BARRON'S

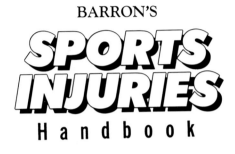

SPORTS
INJURIES
Handbook

BARRON'S
SPORTS INJURIES
H a n d b o o k

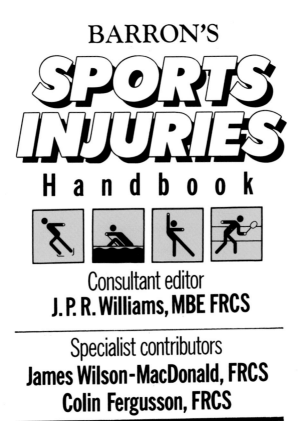

Consultant editor
J. P. R. Williams, MBE FRCS

Specialist contributors
James Wilson-MacDonald, FRCS
Colin Fergusson, FRCS

Barron's
New York

First edition for the United States published 1988 by
Barron's Educational Series, Inc.

All inquiries should be addressed to:
Barron's Educational Series, Inc.
250 Wireless Boulevard
Hauppauge, New York 11788

Library of Congress Catalog Card No. 87-37426

International Standard Book No. 0-8120-5915-8

Library of Congress Cataloging-in-Publication Data

Sports injuries handbook.

Includes index.
1. Sports – Accidents and injuries – Handbooks, manuals,
etc. I. Williams, J.P.R. (John Peter Rhys), 1949-
RD97.S687 1988 617'.1027 87-37426
ISBN 0-8120-5915-8

Editorial Director: Loraine Fergusson
Art Director: Peter Laws
Illustration: Craig Austin, David Ashby
Photography: John Heseltine
Indexer: Susan Ramsey

Printed and bound in Portugal by Printer Portuguesa Lda

The information contained in this book, whilst it has been obtained
from professional medical sources and every care has been taken to
ensure that it is consistent with current medical practice, it is intended
only as a guide to current medical practice in the field of sports injuries
and not as a substitute for the advice of your medical practitioner which
must, on all occasions, be taken promptly following injury.

CONTENTS

Introduction

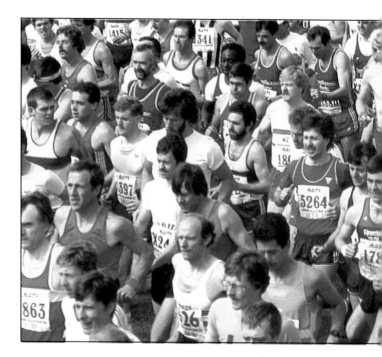

Injury occurs in sports as it does in day to day life. The difference is that sports injuries are avoidable. However, there is still a general shortage of information available to athletes about how to treat various injuries, and it is hoped that the book will help to fill the gap by providing information in an easy to understand form.

Injury prevention begins with the physical evaluation of athletes before they take up a sport. Much is known now about the hazards of each individual sport, and physical deficiencies can be spotted at the beginning of the season and rectified. This is particularly true of the elderly athlete, and is dealt with in **Section One**.

Physical conditioning of the athlete is important to prevent injury. Strength, flexibility, coordination and power are required in different proportions for different sports, and these can only be gained by correct training and pre-sport warming-up exercises. **Section One: Getting Fit** should help you here. In sports such as sailing, riding and jogging, attention to equipment is most important and some advice appears in **Section One: Protective Equipment**.

Most sporting injuries are relatively minor and can be treated by the athlete. In **Section Two: Injuries Guide**,

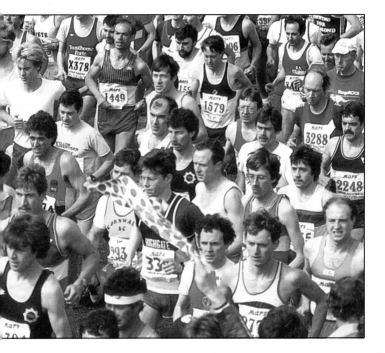

injuries are dealt with according to the part of the body which they affect. You should be able to diagnose an injury and follow the recommended treatment, whether it is a home remedy or an injury that requires medical attention. If in doubt, always ask someone, such as a trainer, physical therapist or doctor, preferably trained in sports medicine. Do not ignore the recommendation of Rest, Ice, Compression, Elevation (RICE, see page 119). Early treatment of many injuries results in a much shorter time off sports and easier return to competition.

Section Four: Sport-Specific Injuries looks at injuries which occur in specific sports and gives advice on changes in technique which may help. It is worth reading the section on your chosen sport to alert you to possible dangers before they lead to injury.

Appendix I at the end of the book explains the meaning of common medical words used by doctors or other medical staff, and finally there is a section on **Sports and Women**.

The book hopes to help you avoid injury in the first place, explain an injury should it occur and give you advice on the best approach to treatment.

Foreword

The past two decades have seen a virtual explosion in athletic participation and in both formal and informal fitness activity. Today, involvement in athletics and fitness starts at a much earlier age and continues well into the late senior years. Fitness, ability, and skill enhancement programs, once designed for only the elite athlete, are now being designed for and used by a much wider audience of athletes.

With the passing of each generation, athletic performance and skill proficiency surpasses that of preceding generations. This causes increased stress on the anatomical and physiological status of the athlete, producing a plethora of overuse injuries, many of which are sport-specific-related. The incidence of overuse injuries can be diminished significantly by methods that improve sports technique, by an increase in the participants' overall level and by the use of proper protective equipment and apparel.

Overzealous fitness and training programs can, in themselves, be harmful to the athlete unless they are set up and carried out by trained, experienced personnel. A proper pre-participation evaluation is also most advisable.

The importance of a proper warm-up, stretching, and cooling down in the prevention of sports injuries must be stressed. Warm-up and stretching are different modalities, and both should be properly performed prior to sports activity. Adequate rest to allow for repair of the athletically stressed tissue is a most important factor in the prevention of injury. The increased occurrence of injury while in fatigued states has been frequently noted.

This handbook of sports injuries presents a panoramic view of the prevention, diagnosis, and treatment of sports injuries in a simple, concise, easy-to-understand manner. The definitions of sports-related terms aids in building a foundation for a better understanding of athletic physical conditions which, in turn, should enhance athletic performance and allow for greater enjoyment and increased fitness.

Dr. Irving V. Glick
Chairman, Sports Medicine Committee USTA
Tournament Physician, U.S. Open
Tournament Physician, Virginia Slims Championships
Tournament Physician, Nabisco Masters Championships
Medical Commission, International Tennis Federation
Team Physician, St. John's University Basketball

SECTION

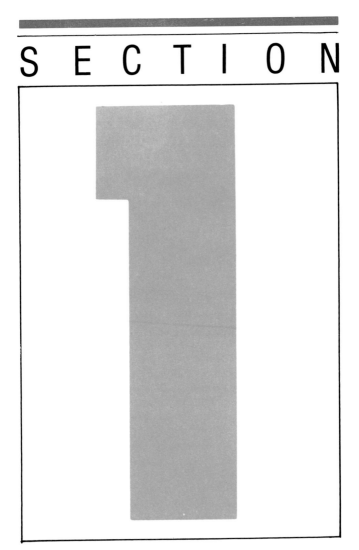

FIT FOR SPORTS
PROTECTIVE EQUIPMENT
GETTING FIT

Fit for Sports

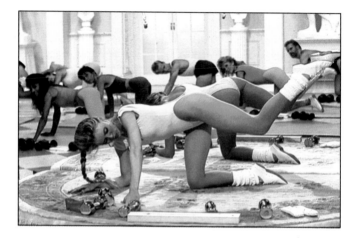

There is good evidence that regular sports lengthen your life-span and make the quality of life more enjoyable. Regular exercise keeps weight down thus diminishing the risks of heart attacks, diabetes and strokes. Depression and other psychiatric illnesses are less common among people who take part in regular sports. Also, the fitter you become, the less likely you are to want to damage your health by smoking, drinking alcohol or taking drugs. Regular sports really means exercise at least twice a week for more than 20 minutes – less is probably not beneficial and injury may be more likely because of the lack of training.

However, it is a mistake to assume that strenuous exercise is the answer for everyone, that the more you do the fitter you will be, or that exercise can cure all ailments. Most sports injuries are avoidable if you cut down on the risk factors by avoiding sports you are not suited to and training and warming up correctly, particularly when taking up a new sport or starting again after a long layoff.

Contraindications

However unfit you are, there will almost always be a sport you can take part in, although some chest and heart diseases may prevent you from playing very active sports. There are no definite rules, and if you are in doubt, you should ask the advice of your doctor. Conditions that need supervision include angina (heart pain); previous heart attack; high blood pressure; atrial fibrillation (irregular pulse); asthma; bronchitis; diseases of the blood vessels; and diseases of the muscles or bones.

Fitness assessment

Anyone over the age of 40 taking up an energetic sport such as squash after a long layoff should arrange to have a fitness assessment of some type. Certain drugs may interfere with sporting activity. If you are in any doubt, ask your doctor.

Medical examination is the simplest form of fitness assessment. Usually includes an ECG (heart tracing) to check that there is no abnormality. Can be done by your doctor.

Sport-specific examination is carried out by trained personnel affiliated with a particular type of sport who can advise on training routines relative to that particular sport. These specialists also give advise on training routines.

Fitness testing

Warning!
All fitness tests such as step tests, bicycle, rowing machine, ergometer or treadmill tests should be done under medical supervision.

Step tests up and down on a standard height of step at a pre-set speed for a given number of minutes, e.g. 30 times per minute for four minutes. The time it takes for the heart to slow to normal pulse rate after the exercise indicates the fitness of the individual. The quicker the heart slows down, the fitter the person.

Bicycle or rowing machine ergometers are set up so that there is a variable resistance to the exercise allowing the workload to be set. As in the step tests, the exercise is performed at a given rate and for a given time. Fitness is assessed by heart rate and the speed with which the heart rate falls. Alternatively, the machines can be used in conjunction with sophisticated apparatus which measures oxygen consumption and hence fitness.

Treadmill tests are commonly used by doctors to assess fitness of patients with heart disease as well as healthy athletes.

Diet

Energy given out by food is measured in calories (kilocalories), and the average requirement is 3,000 calories per day. If you lie in bed all day, you only need 1,500 calories, but if you are mountaineering all day in the cold, you may need 6,000 calories or more.

Carbohydrates are the most important form of energy for the body. They are found in many foods, but particularly in bread, sugar and cereal products. Carbohydrates should form more than half of your calorie intake.

Proteins are the body's building blocks but they are not easily metabolized and the high protein diet traditionally favored by athletes in training is now thought to lead to heart disease and other problems.

Fat is the most concentrated form of energy, but most of the fat eaten is stored in the body and only used as a last resort when other energy stores are used up (in prolonged exercise fat becomes a much more important source of energy). However, you do need a certain amount of fat in your diet because many vitamins are absorbed with it. Generally, vegetable fats (unsaturated fats) are thought to be safer because they lower the incidence of heart disease and strokes.

The training diet

High carbohydrate diets have been shown to be helpful in endurance events such as cross-country skiing or bicycling, but in general specific diet regimes have never been proven to be advantageous – a balanced diet is still best. However, if you are diabetic seek medical advice about diet. Similarly, there is no evidence that vitamins make the slightest difference to performance. A balanced diet provides all the vitamins the body needs.

Precompetition eating

Do not exercise within three to four hours after eating a large meal because much of the blood supply needed for muscular exercise goes to the stomach and intestines during digestion and this may cause a stitch or cramps. Eating glucose or other carbohydrates within an hour or two of an event will weaken you and is detrimental to your performance.

What is fitness?

Fitness is literally the ability to perform your particular sport to your full potential. It has come to mean, however, the improved efficiency of the muscles and cardiovascular system to respond to physical exertion.

Muscle

Muscle has the ability to convert energy into movement. Energy comes from biochemical reactions in the muscle which break down the fuel (e.g., glucose). This conversion is at its most efficient when there is lots of oxygen present (aerobic exercise). However, the body can make energy from fuel without oxygen for a short period of time (up to 40 seconds) but this is less efficient and produces unpleasant by-products (lactic acid) which can cause cramps and stiffness the following day.

Aerobic training

To get more energy more quickly out of your muscles, you need to get more oxygen to your muscles and improve the efficiency with which you use it. In order to do this, you have to practice maintaining exercise at a comfortable level. If you over exert the muscles and demand more energy from them than they can give, they run out of oxygen and start producing energy anaerobically (without oxygen). So, if you are unfit, you need to build up your aerobic stamina gradually. If an exercise begins to hurt, slow down. To maintain fitness you should exercise moderately for at least 20 minutes three times a week.

Anaerobic training

If you are not a athlete, you never require your muscles to produce energy anaerobically. However, an athlete requires all the energy the muscles can provide and with regular training he or she can teach the muscles to efficiently produce energy anaerobically with fewer by-products such as lactic acid. This form of training involves intense exercise for up to one minute followed by either more gentle exercise or complete rest for four to five minutes. The routine should be repeated five or ten times during training sessions.

Smoking

Smoking is the cause of most lung damage. Smoking does not have one beneficial effect on the body and is most inadvisable for any athlete. Not only does it damage the lungs over a number of years, but it also damages the blood vessels and eventually the heart. Even smoking a few cigarettes has a detrimental effect on the body.

The heart

At rest the heart pumps five quarts of blood around the body supplying organs such as the intestines, liver, kidneys and brain. Exercise depends on the output of blood from the heart. This cardiac output is measured by the amount of blood pumped out of the heart every beat, multiplied by the number of heart beats each minute. A large, efficient heart shifts more blood at each pump and during exercise the volume of blood pumped by the heart can increase by up to eight times to 40 quarts of blood per minute. However, an inefficient heart has to pump more frequently to compensate and an unfit person may only be able to pump 25 quarts of blood around the body each minute even when the heart is racing at 180 to 200 beats a minute. Beyond this point the heart becomes inefficient.

A fit person's heart responds to exercise swiftly, and quickly slows down to normal when exercise stops. The improved efficiency of the heart means that at rest a trained athlete has a lower than normal heart rate but during hard exercise the heart can beat at a very high rate without losing efficiency.

Most heart diseases lessen the efficiency of the heart by damaging the muscle of the heart itself.

The lungs

The lungs transfer gases in and out of the body. Oxygen is needed to burn the calories taken in the form of food to produce energy. Carbon dioxide is produced as a by-product of energy production. Blood enters the lungs full of carbon dioxide which is transferred to the air in the lungs and breathed out (exhaled). With the next in-breath (inhalation) oxygen is transferred from the air into the blood and is then taken to the muscles where it is used to burn food and form energy. A fit person has more efficient lungs because more blood passes through them.

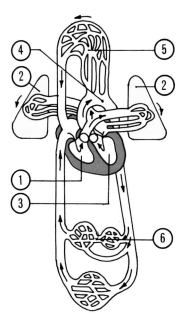

The right side of the heart (1) pumps blood low in oxygen to (2) the lungs. (3) The left side pumps oxygen-rich blood along (4) the aorta to (5) the head and arms and (6) the internal organs.

Blood

Oxygen and carbon dioxide are transported by the blood in the red blood cells. Too few red blood cells (anemia), reduces the amount of oxygen that can be carried, thus reducing fitness. Anemia is rare in men, more common in women (see **Appendix II: Sports and Women**). Smoking also reduces the ability of the blood to carry oxygen.

Heat loss

All chemical reactions produce heat, and the production of energy in the body is no exception. The fitter a person is, the better his or her body becomes at losing this excess heat during exercise. Heat is lost in three ways. When you sweat, the moisture evaporates and the surface of the skin cools; when you breathe heat from the body is expelled with each exhalation; and the blood supply to the skin can increase up to 50 times during exercise giving off much of its heat. The body of a fit person is able to stand a much higher temperature. Salt and water losses may be high in sports of long duration and may need replacement.

Protective Equipment

Footwear

Many sporting injuries could be prevented by using correct footwear. Go for the best you can afford, and ask advice about which type of shoe is most suitable for your sport. The road running shoe in the picture could cause an injury if used for playing squash, badminton or tennis because the wide-based sole makes it too stable for the rolling and twisting the foot needs to do during racquet sports. Similarly the aerobic shoe is perfect for on-the-spot jogging and dancing on a flat floor but would be completely unsuitable for the rigors of road or cross-country running. Make sure that the uppers are made of a natural fiber such as leather, canvas or suede. When buying footwear, use the socks you intend to wear in the future.

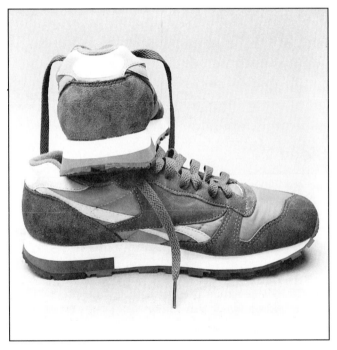

Road running shoe with a thick, padded sole which widens out at the base offers extra stability. These shoes are cut away at the back which helps to prevent achilles' tendinitis.

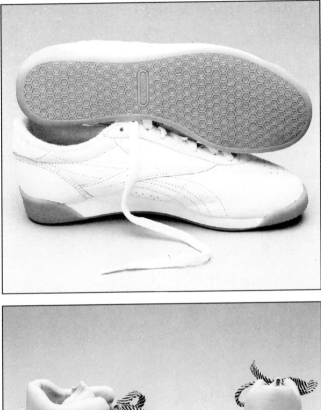

Aerobic shoes (top) need to be lightweight with a flexible sole whereas the walking boot (below) must give the ankle as much support as possible and have a sole thick enough to deal with rough terrain.

Helmets and goggles

Injuries to the head are potentially the most life-threatening and no expense should be spared when buying properly fitting headgear. A helmet that has saved you once from a bad fall or blow should be replaced because it is likely to have been weakened.

In contrast, eye protection is relatively inexpensive. Unfortunately, many people simply forget to protect their eyes or find goggles for games such as squash, unacceptable. This is a risky attitude because an eye injury can be devastating – a broken leg usually heals, a blow to the eye may lead to blindness.

Skiing goggles (top) protect against reflected glare which can damage the eyes; squash goggles (left) have no lenses but prevent the squash ball from impacting into the eye socket; and swimming goggles (right) of this variety protect the delicate lining of the eyes from chlorine and salt in the water.

A helmet (below left) with the additional protection of a face guard of coated metal or plastic protects the player's face against all but the severest impacts. A riding helmet (below right) should be chosen in preference to the standard hat which offers very little protection in a fall.

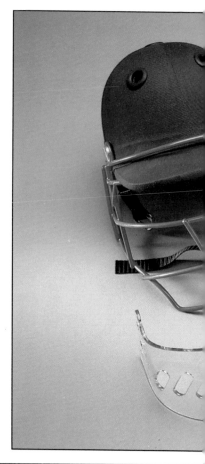

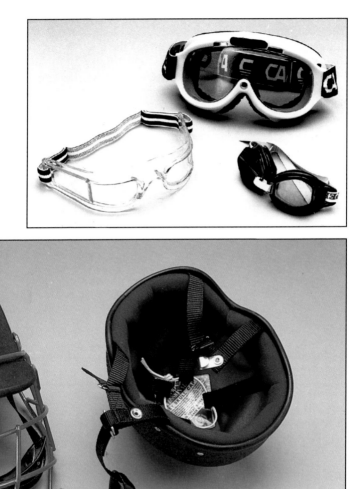

Shields, pads and gloves

The equipment on the previous page protects you against unlikely but disasterous injury whereas the body armor on this page protects you against inevitable injury and much of it is regarded as an essential part of the sport. However, it is worth keeping up to date with what is available because safety and comfort standards are being constantly improved.

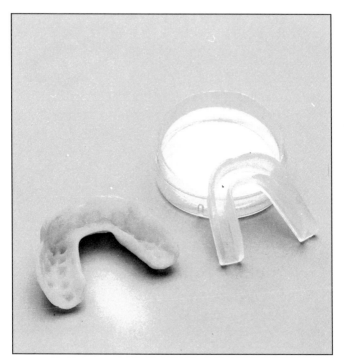

A custom-made gum shield (left) is more comfortable to wear, stays in place and offers the best protection against blows to the mouth. However, it is very much more expensive than a standard gum shield. To use one of these, soak the shield in boiling water to soften the plastic, place it over your upper set of teeth and bite it hard into place. You may have to repeat the operation a few times until it is comfortable and stays in place when you open your mouth.

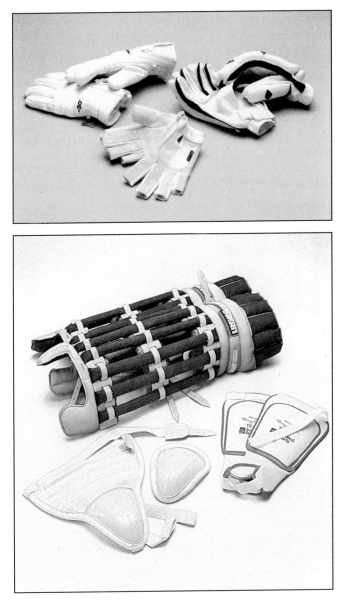

Hand protection against the cold for skiing (left); blows to the thumb (right); and rope burns for sailing (center).

Body armor for shins in hockey (top) and soccer (right) plus genital and lower abdominal protection for baseball.

Safe watersports

All watersports are potentially dangerous. Even if you are a competent swimmer you should wear a buoyancy aid for any watersports including waterskiing, windsurfing and canoeing, because a fall or a blow may knock you unconscious. A non-swimmer participating in watersports of any kind must be protected by a life preserver. It is always safest to participate in watersports with another person, but if you do go alone, always let someone know where you are going and when you expect to be back.

You must also be careful to protect yourself against the cold. A stiff wind blowing on wet clothing can chill the

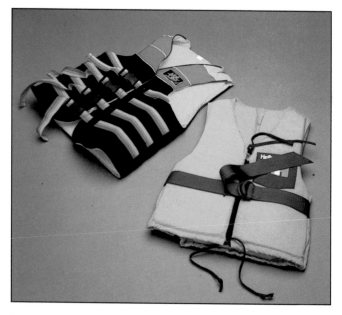

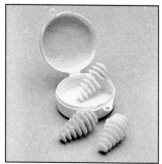

Buoyancy aids can be fitted (above left) for waterskiing and windsurfing to make them more streamlined, or standard for dingy sailing (above right). Ear plugs (left) may offer some protection for swimming, but should never be worn for diving because water pressure may force them into the ears.

body at an alarming rate and may cause hypothermia, a potentially life-threatening condition when the temperature of the body drops rapidly. For windsurfing and waterskiing a wetsuit offers good protection. When sailing, a great deal of heat can be lost from the legs and head – it is not enough to wear water- and windproof clothing on the upper body alone.

You may also need to protect against heat and sunburn. A great deal of the sun's rays are reflected up off the surface of the water doubling the sunburn rate, so wear a waterproof sunblock cream on all exposed areas.

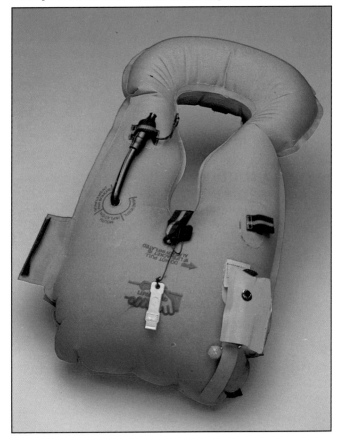

A life preserver is an expensive piece of equipment, but it can be inflated in seconds and keep even an unconscious person afloat in the correct position.

Getting Fit

There are two reasons for exercising outside your sport. The first is to prevent injury and the second is to improve your performance in your sport.

Exercise of this type falls into three main categories: stretching exercises to improve flexibility; power exercises to increase strength and muscle bulk; and fitness exercises to make the body more efficient. The exercises on the following pages can be used in two ways to avoid injury, either as a warm-up routine before sports, or as general fitness and suppleness exercises.

Warming up

Moderate exercise may not require much warming up beforehand – for example, jogging is often used as a warm up exercise in itself, and games such as squash and tennis include a practice which gets the muscles warm and raises the pulse rate. However, the more strenuous the exercise, the more time you must set aside for the warm up. Age should also affect the time you spend on the exercises – the older you are, the longer the warm up should be.

Training routine

If you have not played any sport for a number of years a quick warm up is not going to be enough. You need to work out a proper training routine, one month of training for every year that you were inactive. Such a routine could easily be made up from the following exercises along with a sensible jogging and running program.

Do not be tempted to overexert yourself or you will become exhausted, stiff and dispirited. For your jogging program begin with a stiff walk for 20 minutes. After a few days incorporate periods of jogging, slowing down to a walk again if you become too out of breath. You will soon find you are jogging for more of the 20 minutes than you are walking. Once you can jog comfortably, build up the time and distance.

Complementary exercise

The nature of many sports means that you can only improve your performance up to a particular level through participation. For example, a swimmer can greatly increase his or her stamina with distance swimming, but muscle bulk increase is limited. Weight training can greatly improve the swimmer's speed and efficiency by developing powerful arm, chest and leg muscles. The opposite problem affects the sprinter. A 60-meter dash does not build up lung efficiency and stamina. The sprinter becomes more efficient at the sport by improving stamina through aerobic training of various types.

Stretching Exercises

The importance of warming up cannot be over-emphasized because cold, tight muscles are more likely to be injured. The amateur athlete often ignores the warm up even though it can be completed in a few minutes. However, as you become fitter you can increase the time spent on the warm up. Do the exercises smoothly, increasing your range and the vigor of the movement as you feel the large muscle groups limbering up. Never force a movement – gradually push yourself a little further on each repetition. As well as loosening and limbering, these exercises raise the pulse rate in readiness for the subsequent power exercises.

Arm stretch

To improve shoulder mobility, swing your arms up keeping the upper arms as close to your head as possible. Swing the arms down behind you, pressing them back as far as you can until your shoulder blades touch, then down to the starting position again. Do the exercise in reverse. Repeat in both directions ten times. This exercise puts the shoulder girdle through its complete range of movement.

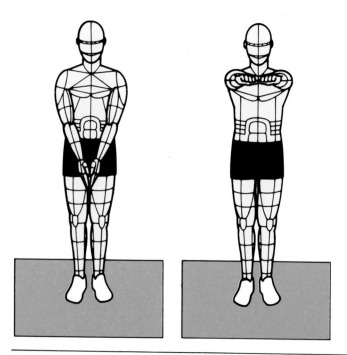

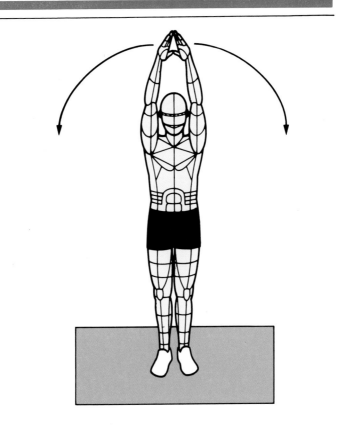

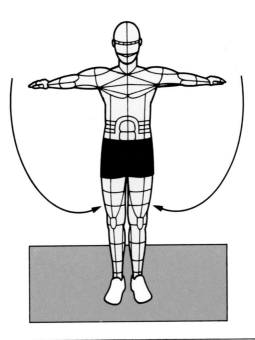

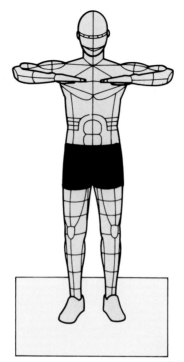

Waist twist

To do this exercise correctly,
it is important to keep your
hips facing forward so that
you are moving just your
torso. This is easier if you
tuck your pelvis under by
tensing your buttock muscles.
Hold your arms at shoulder
height and twist to one side
extending the leading arm to
increase your swing. Swing
back to the front and
smoothly around in the other
direction. Do ten repetitions,
gradually increasing the speed
of the turn. Over the space of
two weeks, work up to 20
repetitions.

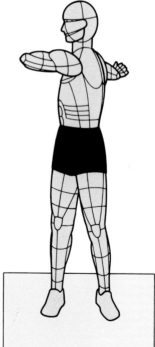

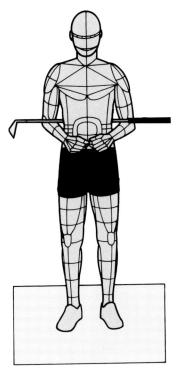

Back turn

This exercise is more effective if you hook your arms around something like a broomstick or golf club. Stand with your feet apart, knees relaxed, and rotate your back as far as it will comfortably go. Let your hip move with you and turn your head in the direction of the twist. Do ten repetitions working up to 20 as your back becomes more mobile.

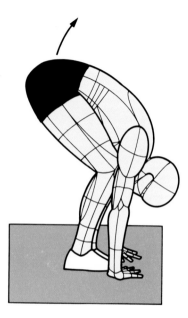

Hamstring stretch

Place your hands on the floor
with your knees bent and
your chest resting on your
upper legs. Gently straighten
the knees trying to keep your
hands on the floor. Do not
force this exercise. Repeat
twelve times.

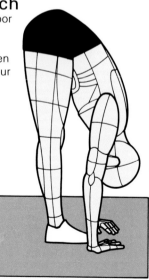

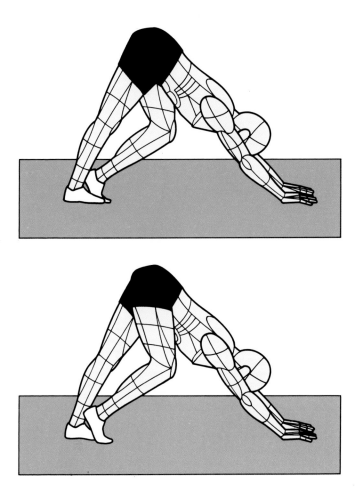

Achilles' tendon stretch
With hands flat on the floor
and back straight, press one
heel downward relaxing the
opposite knee. Do the same
with the opposite heel setting
up a rhythmical and steady
treading action. Continue until
the legs begin to feel tired.

Waist stretch

Stand with feet apart, knees relaxed and pull down to one side reaching out with the leading arm. Keep your body as upright as possible and do not let your shoulder twist forward. You should feel the stretch in muscles up the side of the body. Pull down five times to the right, then five times to the left coming to the upright position between each pull.

Combination stretch

Lunge forward with the right foot directly beneath the knee. Keeping your trailing leg straight, press the hips gently toward the floor until you feel the pull in the trailing leg. Now raise your buttocks and straighten the front leg as much as you can keeping your chest near your upper leg. Press both heels into the ground. Don't force the knee straight – as flexibility increases this will happen naturally. Repeat three times building up to ten over the space of six weeks.

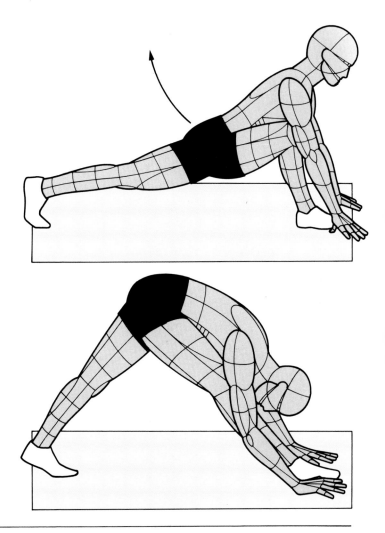

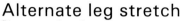

Alternate leg stretch

Place your hands on your
knee to support your upper
body, then press forward and
downward. Keeping your feet
on the same spot, twist
around and push downward
in the opposite direction.
Repeat five times each way.
As flexibility increases you
can bring your trailing leg
back as you come into the
upright position, then lunge
forward with the other leg.

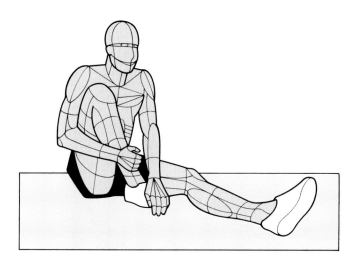

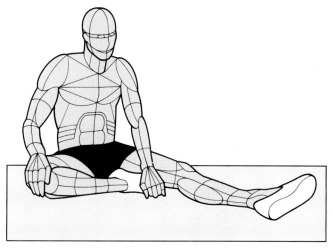

Hip stretch

Sit on the floor with one leg extended and pull the other foot up toward the center of your body. Holding your foot with one hand, press your knee down toward the floor and hold for a count of ten. At first the range of movement will be slight, but within six weeks there will be a noticeable improvement in mobility as the adductor muscle stretches out.

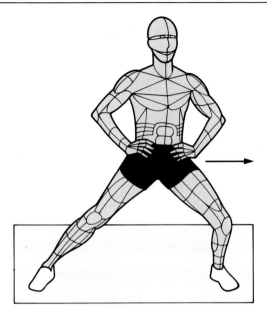

Adductor lunge

Keeping your back straight and your buttocks tight, lunge sideways until you feel the pull in the groin, then swing across and lunge in the opposite direction. Repeat ten times. As mobility increases, bend your knee further to give the adductor more pull.

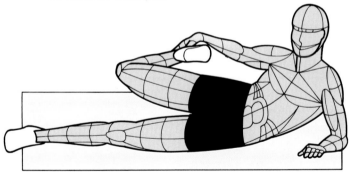

Quads stretch

Lie propped up with one elbow on the floor, grab your ankle and pull your foot up behind you. You should feel the pull at the front of your upper leg. As flexibility increases, roll gently onto your back with your heel held up against your buttock and hold for a count of ten. Repeat with the other leg.

Power Exercises

Different sports build up different muscle groups, but by including the following power exercises in your warm-up routine, you can maintain the condition of the other muscles in the body. Strong muscles in the back and abdomen prevent many back injuries because the stomach muscles take a large proportion of the strain when lifting and help to brace the spine. All the power exercises will raise your pulse rate, but the star jumps and jumping jacks can be used to push it up to training level. Alternatively, use them to maintain fitness if you only play sports once a week. They are vigorous exercises – make sure you have warmed up and stretched all the other muscles before doing them.

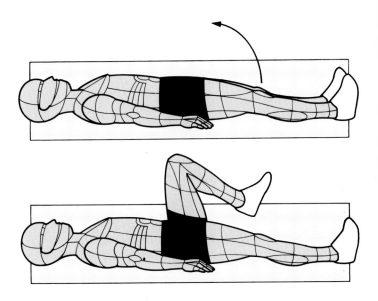

Alternate knee raise

A gentle start to abdominal strengthening exercises. Lie down and press the small of your back onto the floor, pulling your stomach muscles inward. Raise one knee to the count of five, lower it to the count of five, then raise and lower the other leg. Repeat five times with each leg.

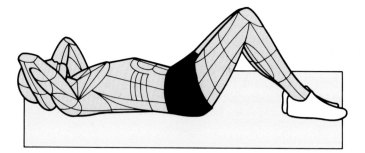

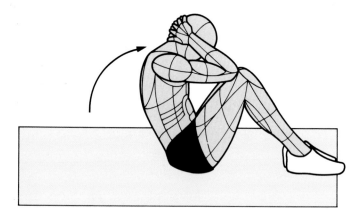

Sit-ups

Place your feet apart and flat
on the floor. Support your
neck muscles by clasping
your hands behind your head.
Hold your stomach muscles in
and sit up. Start with three
controlled sit-ups, and when
you can do these with ease,
increase the number. Some
sort of padding under the
buttocks prevents bruising of
the coccyx.

Figure-U sit-ups

You may not be able to
achieve this until you have
strengthened your stomach
muscles for a few weeks
using the other exercises. The
starting position is the same
as for a regular sit-up, but the
knees and elbows should
come together on one
movement. Hold the position
for a count of three then
come down again. Start with
three and increase the
number gradually.

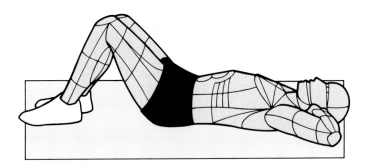

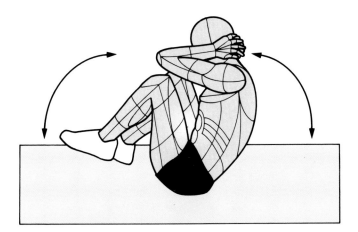

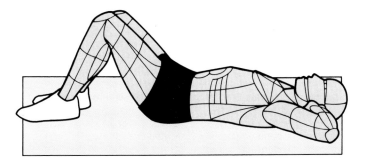

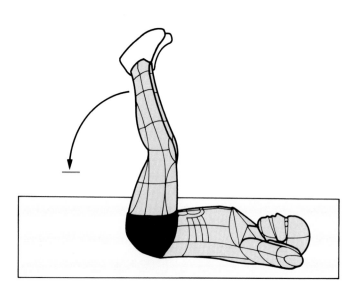

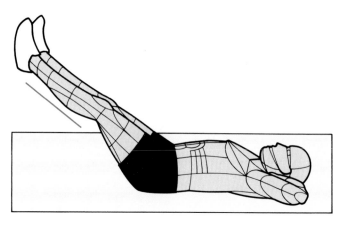

Leg lowering

This strengthens not only the abdominal muscles but also the quads at the top of the leg. Pressing the small of your back onto the floor, start with legs held high, knees slightly bent, then lower them slowly. As soon as you feel the small of your back arching off the ground, raise your legs again. As your strength increases you will be able to get your legs nearer to the floor without your back coming up. Build up to ten.

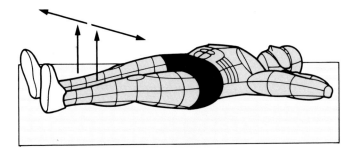

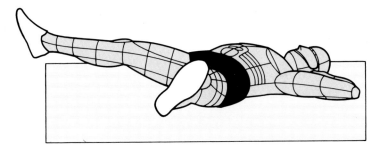

Low scissors

Lie on the floor and raise your legs to a height where you can keep the small of your back on the floor. Holding this position, open and close your legs for four scissor movements, lower and relax. Repeat. As with the previous exercise, the stronger your stomach muscles become, the lower you can hold your legs. Build up the number of scissor movements.

Squat thrusts

It is important to complete the full range of movement in this vigorous exercise. Pump your knees forward and back increasing the speed as your strength increases. Start with five and build up.

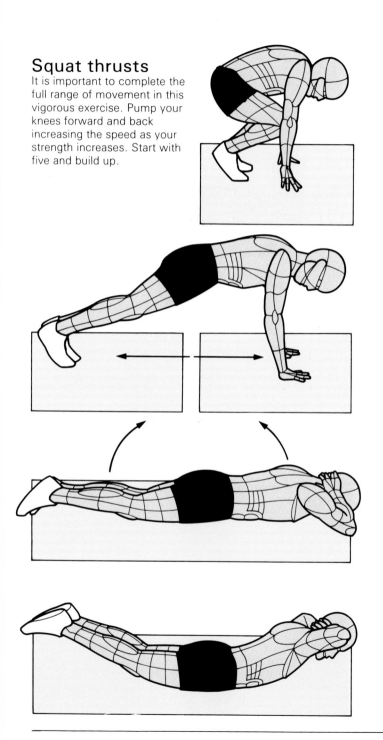

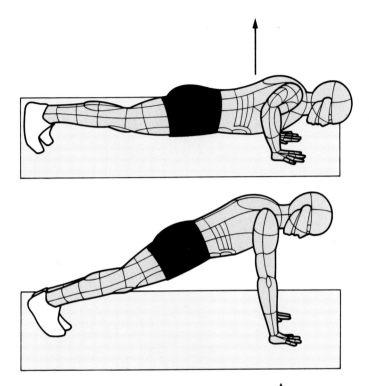

◀ Back arch raises

These supple and strengthen the back muscles. Lie on your front and place your hands behind your neck. Pull your shoulders and legs off the floor and hold for a count of five. Begin with five and increase the ten.

Push-ups ▲

These should be controlled and accurate. Start with two until you really master the knack of keeping your legs and back absolutely straight as you pivot on your toes. Keep your hands directly under your shoulders at first, and when you can do ten push-ups with comparative ease, move your hands further outward for extra benefit.

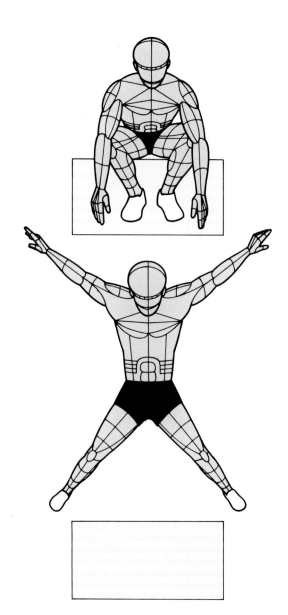

Star jumps

Start in a squatting position, then spring as high as you can to get your arms and legs into the star position before landing in the squat again. This exercise needs some practice but the height of your jump will increase. Start with two good ones, then build up to ten or fifteen over a space of a few weeks.

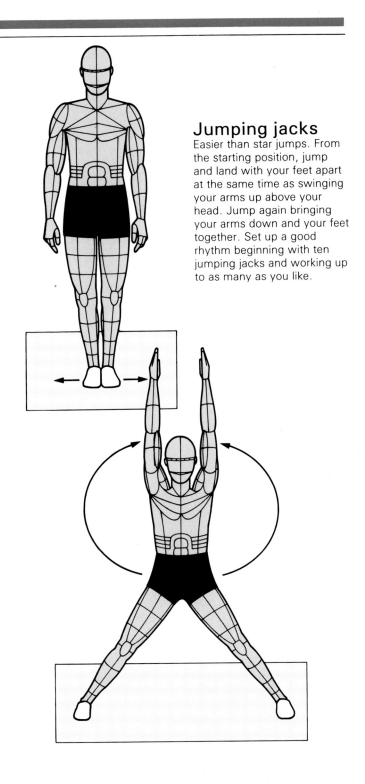

Jumping jacks

Easier than star jumps. From the starting position, jump and land with your feet apart at the same time as swinging your arms up above your head. Jump again bringing your arms down and your feet together. Set up a good rhythm beginning with ten jumping jacks and working up to as many as you like.

Pulse Rate

Working pulse rate

To get the best from aerobic exercise, you should keep your heart working at between 70% to 80% of the rate your heart can beat at maximum. This top rate decreases by one beat each minute for every year of your life. You can check your target pulse rate on the chart below.

Take your pulse after a few minutes of hard exercise (count it for 15 seconds and multiply by four), and you will be able to see if you are working too hard or not hard enough.

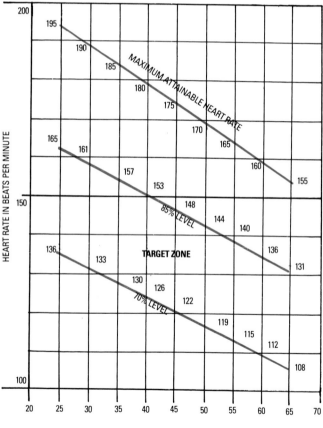

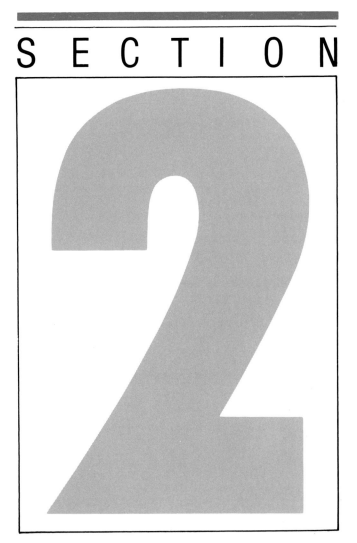

S E C T I O N

INJURIES GUIDE

How to Use this Section

Pages 50-61 form an anatomical guide to parts of the body commonly injured during sports. (1) Find the page that applies to your injury. (2) The illustrations show some useful anatomical details as well as areas of possible trouble. (3) Find the area which most accurately matches your pain, then (4) look the number up on the list. (5) Here you will find a page number referring you to the part of the book concerned with your injury.

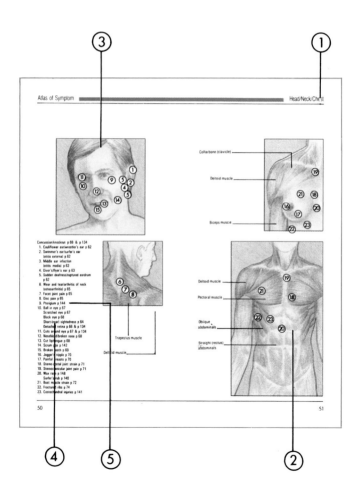

Collarbone (clavicle)

Deltoid muscle

Biceps muscle

Concussion/knockout p 69 & p 134
1. Cauliflower ear/wrestler's ear p 62
2. Swimmer's ear/surfer's ear (otitis external) p 62
3. Middle ear infection (otitis media) p 63
4. Diver's/flyer's ear p 63
5. Sudden deafness/ruptured eardrum p 62
6. Wear and tear/arthritis of neck (osteoarthritis) p 65
7. Facet joint pain p 65
8. Disc pain p 65
9. Pterigium p 144
10. Ball in eye p 67
    Scratched eye p 67
    Black eye p 68
    Short-sight/near sightedness p 64
    Detached retina p 66 & p 134
11. Cuts around eye p 67 & p 134
12. Nosebleed/broken nose p 68
13. Cut lip/tongue p 68
14. Scrum gum p 142
15. Broken tooth p 68
16. Jogger's nipple p 70
17. Painful breasts p 70
18. Sternoclavicular joint strain p 71
19. Sternoclavicular joint pain p 71
20. Wax rash p 148
    Surfer's nub p 148
21. Bust muscle strain p 72
22. Fractured ribs p 74
23. Costochondral injuries p 141

Trapezius muscle

Deltoid muscle

Deltoid muscle

Pectoral muscle

Oblique abdominals

Straight (rectus) abdominals

50

51

48

(6) Once you have turned to the correct page, you will find a common name and often a medical equivalent (7). If the word has a symbol ✪ beside it, this means it is an acute condition – one that happens suddenly rather than gradually. (8) The first column helps to confirm your diagnosis by giving specific symptoms and an explanation of why the condition has occurred. (9) The second column tells you what to do, how to treat the condition and how to prevent it happening again. (10) Illustrations throughout the text clarify certain points.

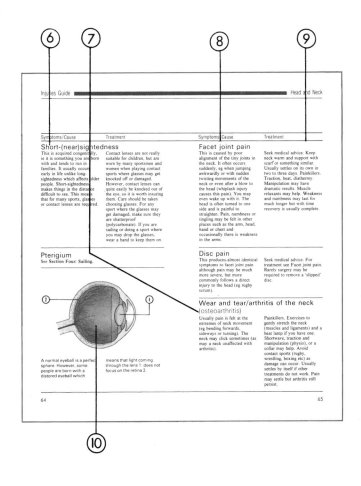

⑥ ⑦ ⑧ ⑨

Injuries Guide ▬▬▬▬▬▬▬▬▬▬▬▬▬▬▬▬▬▬▬▬▬▬▬▬▬▬ Head and Neck

Symptoms/Cause	Treatment	Symptoms/Cause	Treatment
Short-(near)sightedness This is acquired congenitally, ie it is something you are born with and tends to run in families. It usually occurs early in life unlike long-sightedness which affects older people. Short-sightedness makes things in the distance difficult to see. This means that for many sports, glasses or contact lenses are required.	Contact lenses are not really suitable for children, but are worn by many sportsmen and women when playing contact sports where glasses may get knocked off or damaged. However, contact lenses can quite easily be knocked out of the eye, so it is worth insuring them. Care should be taken choosing glasses. For any sport where the glasses may get damaged, make sure they are shatterproof (polycarbonate). If you are sailing or doing a sport where you may drop the glasses, wear a band to keep them on.	**Facet joint pain** This is caused by poor alignment of the tiny joints in the neck. It often occurs suddenly, eg when jumping awkwardly or with sudden twisting movements of the neck or even after a blow to the head (whiplash injury causes this pain). You may even wake up with it. The head is often turned to one side and is painful to straighten. Pain, numbness or tingling may be felt in other places such as the arm, head, hand or chest and occasionally there is weakness in the arms.	Seek medical advice. Keep neck warm and support with scarf or something similar. Usually settles on its own in two to three days. Painkillers. Traction, heat, diathermy. Manipulation may have dramatic results. Muscle relaxants may help. Weakness and numbness may last for much longer but with time recovery is usually complete.
Pterigium See Section Four: Sailing.		**Disc pain** This produces almost identical symptoms to facet joint pain although pain may be much more severe, but more commonly follows a direct injury to the head (eg rugby scrum).	Seek medical advice. For treatment see Facet joint pain. Rarely surgery may be required to remove a 'slipped' disc.
		Wear and tear/arthritis of the neck (osteoarthritis) Usually pain is felt at the extremes of neck movement (eg bending forwards, sideways or turning). The neck may click sometimes (as may a neck unaffected by arthritis).	Painkillers. Exercises to gently stretch the neck (muscles and ligaments) and a heat lamp if you have one. Shortwave, traction and manipulation (physio), or a collar may help. Avoid contact sports (rugby, wrestling, boxing etc) as damage can occur. Usually settles by itself if other treatments do not work. Pain may settle but arthritis still persist.
A normal eyeball is a perfect sphere. However, some people are born with a distorted eyeball which	means that light coming through the lens 1. does not focus on the retina 2.		

64 · 65

⑩

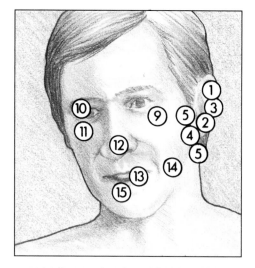

1. Cauliflower ear/wrestler's ear, p.62
2. Swimmer's ear/surfer's ear
   (otitis externa), p.62
3. Middle ear infection
   (otitis media), p.63
4. Diver's/flyer's ear, p.63
5. Sudden deafness/ruptured eardrum, p.62
6. Wear and tear/arthritis of neck
   (osteoarthritis), p.65
7. Facet joint pain, p.65
8. Disc pain, p.65
9. Pterigium, p.144
10. Ball in eye, p.67
    Scratched eye, p.67
    Black eye, p.68
    Nearsightedness, p.64
    Detached retina, p.66 & p.134
11. Cuts around eye, p.67 & p.134
12. Nosebleed/broken nose, p.68
13. Cut lip/tongue, p.68
14. Concussion/knockout, p.69 & p.134
15. Broken tooth, p.69
16. Jogger's nipple, p.70
17. Painful breasts, p.70
18. Sterno-costal joint strain, p.71
19. Sternoclavicular joint pain, p.71
20. Wax rash, p.148
21. Bust muscle strain, p.72
22. Fractured ribs, p.74
23. Surfer's rub, p.148

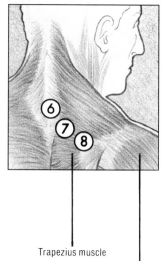

Trapezius muscle

Deltoid muscle

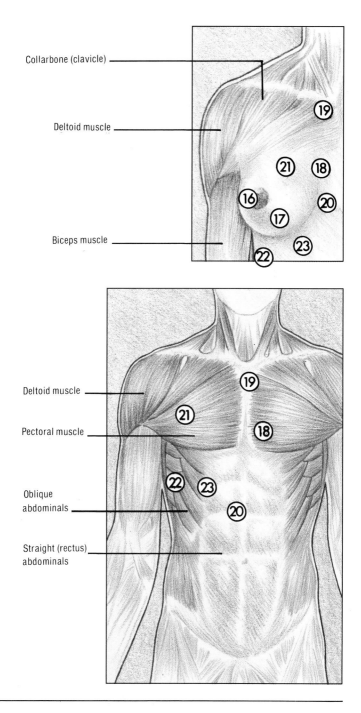

Collarbone (clavicle)

Deltoid muscle

Biceps muscle

Deltoid muscle

Pectoral muscle

Oblique abdominals

Straight (rectus) abdominals

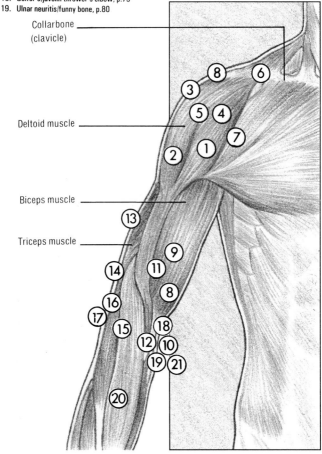

Collarbone
(clavicle)

Deltoid muscle

Biceps muscle

Triceps muscle

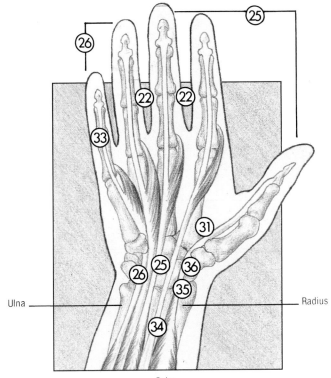

Ulna

Radius

Palm

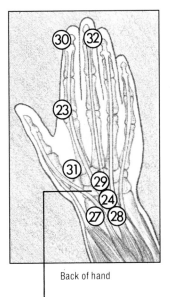

Back of hand

Wrist joint

1. Ligament strain, p.86
2. Bowler's back, p.87
3. Upper back pain, p.87
4. Shoulder-blade rub, p.88
5. Gymnast's back, p.87
6. Coccygitis (coccydynia), p.88
7. Blow to flank, p.88

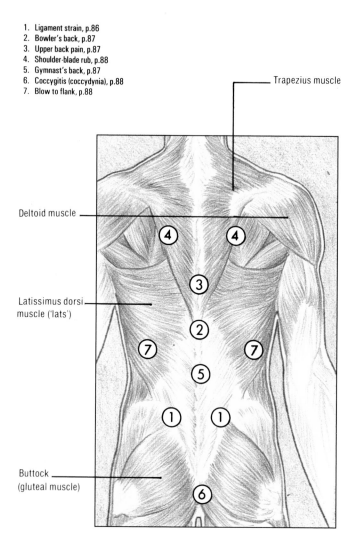

Trapezius muscle

Deltoid muscle

Latissimus dorsi
muscle ('lats')

Buttock
(gluteal muscle)

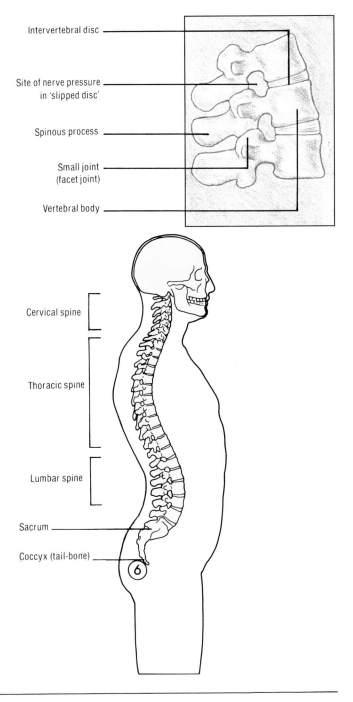

Intervertebral disc

Site of nerve pressure
in 'slipped disc'

Spinous process

Small joint
(facet joint)

Vertebral body

Cervical spine

Thoracic spine

Lumbar spine

Sacrum

Coccyx (tail-bone)

⑥

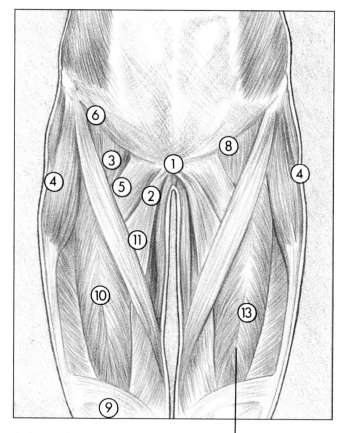

1. Soccer player's groin
   (osteitis pubis symphysis), p.89
2. Adductor strain, p.89
3. High knee hip pain, p.89
4. Trochanteric bursa, p.90
5. Arthritis/hip joint pain, p.90
6. Avulsion fracture, p.90
7. Blow to genitals (men), p.91
8. Hernia (rupture), p.150
9. Quads insertion pull, p.92
10. Quads muscle pull, p.92
11. Adductor muscle strain, p.93
12. Hamstring sprains, p.93
13. Quads injury, p.93

Quadriceps
(quads) muscles

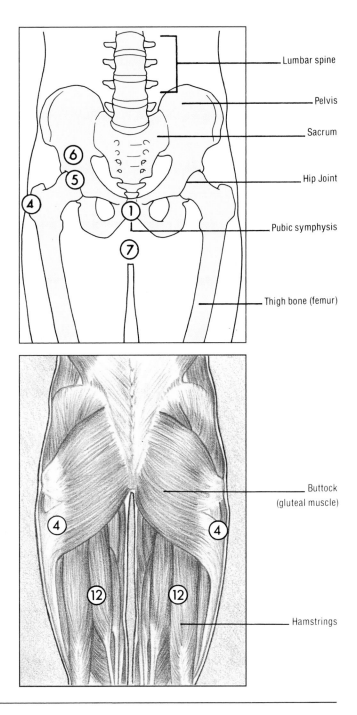

Lumbar spine

Pelvis

Sacrum

Hip Joint

Pubic symphysis

Thigh bone (femur)

Buttock
(gluteal muscle)

Hamstrings

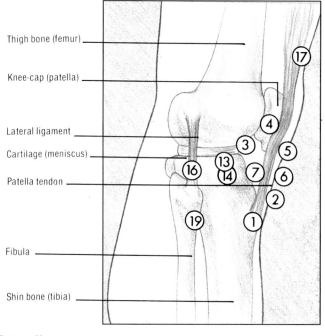

Thigh bone (femur)

Knee-cap (patella)

Lateral ligament

Cartilage (meniscus)

Patella tendon

Fibula

Shin bone (tibia)

Fracture, p.99
Slow swelling/rapid swelling, p.94
Fracture of shin bone, p.105

1. Osgood Schlatter's disease, p.94
2. Housemaid's knee, p.95
3. Teenager's knee
   (osteochondritis dissecans), p.95
4. Kneecap pain
   (patello-femoral pain syndrome), p.95
5. Lower kneecap pain, p.96
6. Jumper's knee (patella tendinitis), p.96
7. Hoffa's syndrome, p.96
8. Hamstring bursa (semimembranosus bursa),
   p.96
9. Baker's cyst, p.97
10. Biceps bursa, p.97
11. Fascia lata strain/iliotibial tract pain, p.97
12. Adductor avulsion, p.97
13. Cartilage (meniscal) injury, p.98
14. Cartilage ligament injury, p.99
15. Medial ligament injury, p.100
16. Lateral ligament strain/rupture, p.101
    Unstable knee/cruciate ligament rupture,
    p.101
17. Quads injury, p.93
18. Dislocated kneecap, p.99
19. Nerve injury, p.101
20. Anterior compartment pain, p.102
21. Shin splints, p.102

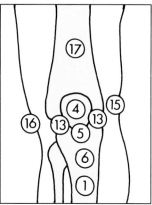

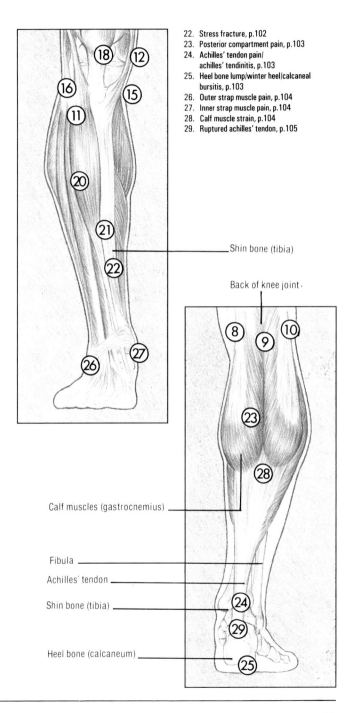

22. Stress fracture, p.102
23. Posterior compartment pain, p.103
24. Achilles' tendon pain/
    achilles' tendinitis, p.103
25. Heel bone lump/winter heel/calcaneal
    bursitis, p.103
26. Outer strap muscle pain, p.104
27. Inner strap muscle pain, p.104
28. Calf muscle strain, p.104
29. Ruptured achilles' tendon, p.105

Shin bone (tibia)

Back of knee joint

Calf muscles (gastrocnemius)

Fibula

Achilles' tendon

Shin bone (tibia)

Heel bone (calcaneum)

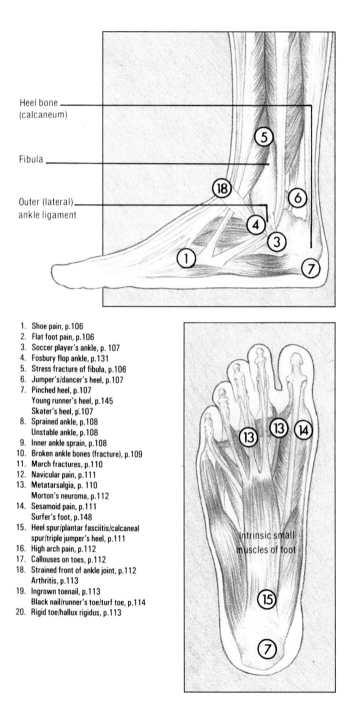

Heel bone (calcaneum)

Fibula

Outer (lateral) ankle ligament

1. Shoe pain, p.106
2. Flat foot pain, p.106
3. Soccer player's ankle, p. 107
4. Fosbury flop ankle, p.131
5. Stress fracture of fibula, p.106
6. Jumper's/dancer's heel, p.107
7. Pinched heel, p.107
   Young runner's heel, p.145
   Skater's heel, p.107
8. Sprained ankle, p.108
   Unstable ankle, p.108
9. Inner ankle sprain, p.108
10. Broken ankle bones (fracture), p.109
11. March fractures, p.110
12. Navicular pain, p.111
13. Metatarsalgia, p. 110
    Morton's neuroma, p.112
14. Sesamoid pain, p.111
    Surfer's foot, p.148
15. Heel spur/plantar fasciitis/calcaneal
    spur/triple jumper's heel, p.111
16. High arch pain, p.112
17. Callouses on toes, p.112
18. Strained front of ankle joint, p.112
    Arthritis, p.113
19. Ingrown toenail, p.113
    Black nail/runner's toe/turf toe, p.114
20. Rigid toe/hallux rigidus, p.113

Intrinsic small muscles of foot

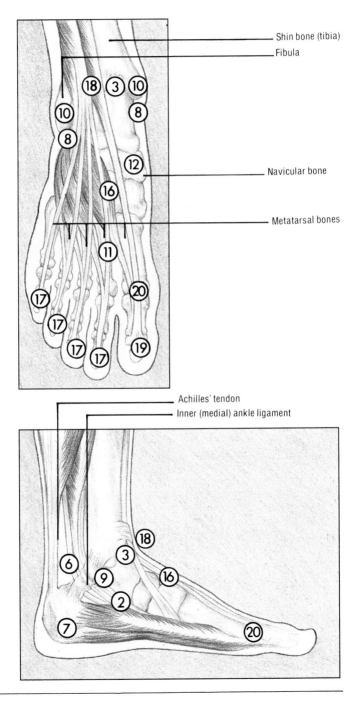

Shin bone (tibia)
Fibula

Navicular bone

Metatarsal bones

Achilles' tendon
Inner (medial) ankle ligament

Head and Neck

Symptoms/Cause	Treatment

Cauliflower ear/wrestler's ear

Condition caused either by repeated injury to the outer soft parts of the ear, or a single injury. Blood accumulates between the gristly part of the ear and the skin. Common in football, boxing, judo and wrestling.

After injury apply compression as soon as possible with ice. Drainage of the blood with a needle by a doctor usually makes the ear less painful and may prevent permanent disfigurement. Plastic surgery is rarely needed. Prevent by wearing a helmet or sweat band.

Swimmer's ear/surfer's ear
(otitis externa)

An infection in the canal between the eardrum and the outer ear. Pain is usually felt in the ear canal itself and around the opening of the canal. Hurts to chew. Ear feels blocked. There may be a discharge of pus or similar material. It is usually caused by the ear being continually wet or by chlorine in swimming pools.

Seek medical advice. Antibiotics. Ear drops are usually very effective but infections can sometimes persist. Make sure ears are dried properly after swimming or other sports, or after bathing to avoid this problem. Ear plugs may prevent it. You may need to stop swimming until the infection has healed.

✪ Sudden deafness/ruptured eardrum

Sudden loud noise in ear accompanied by pain and sometimes dizziness (part of the ear controls balance). Caused by sudden rupture of the eardrum, usually occurs due to sudden pressure change, e.g. loud bang from a gun, underwater diving or high diving.

Keep ear dry. Sometimes requires surgical repair of the very fine membrane of the eardrum, although the drum may repair spontaneously. Ear protection should always be worn while shooting. Avoid swimming until cleared by your doctor.

Symptoms/Cause	Treatment

Middle ear infection (otitis media)

The most serious of the ear infections, caused by infection deep within the ear, it often follows a cold or sore throat. Pain may be severe, and in children it may be felt in other places, e.g. the stomach. Rarely is there a discharge from the ear. Occasionally dizziness and fever.

Seek medical advice. Antibiotics are usually necessary to cure the infection and prevent further spread. Painkillers may be necessary. Occasionally, if infection persists, further treatment is necessary. Avoid swimming until infection subsides. Seek medical advice before flying or scuba diving.

Diver's/flyer's ear

Caused by mucus in the middle ear due to infection. Hearing may be reduced and flying or diving may cause pain or unusual noises in the ear.

If ear pops, hold nose and blow out hard with your mouth shut. This equalizes the pressure inside the ear with that outside. Try chewing gum (but not while swimming). Nasal decongestants should clear the ear, but avoid flying and diving if possible until it heals.

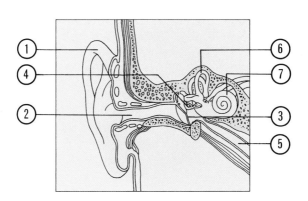

The outer ear is the pinna (1) and ear canal (2). The middle ear is the eardrum (3), three auditory ossicles (miniature bones) (4), and the Eustachian tube (5). The inner ear contains the cochlea (6), and semi-circular canals (7).

Symptoms / Cause	Treatment

Nearsightedness

This is acquired congenitally: it is something you are born with and tends to run in families. It usually occurs early in life unlike farsightedness which affects older people. Nearsightedness makes things in the distance difficult to see. This means that for many sports, glasses or contact lenses are required.

Contact lenses are not really suitable for children, but are worn by many athletes when playing contact sports where glasses may get knocked off or damaged. However, contact lenses can quite easily be knocked out of the eye, so it is worth insuring them. Care should be taken choosing glasses. For any sport where the glasses may get damaged, make sure they are shatterproof (polycarbonate). If you are sailing or doing a sport where you may drop the glasses, wear a band to keep them on.

Pterigium

See **Section Four: Sailing**.

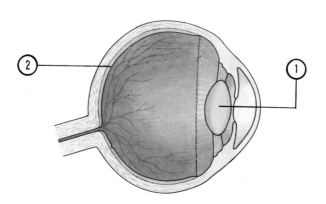

Nearsightedness (see above) occurs when light rays entering the eyeball through the lens (1) do not focus on the retina (2).

Symptoms/Cause	Treatment

Facet joint pain

This is caused by poor alignment of the tiny joints in the neck. It often occurs suddenly, e.g. when jumping awkwardly or with sudden twisting movements of the neck or even after a blow to the head (whiplash injury causes this pain). You may even wake up with it. The head is often turned to one side and is painful to straighten. Pain, numbness or tingling may be felt in other places such as the arm, head, hand or chest and occasionally there is weakness in the arms.

Seek medical advice. Keep neck warm and support with scarf or something similar. Usually subsides on its own in two to three days. Painkillers. Traction, heat, diathermy. Manipulation may have dramatic results. Muscle relaxants may help. Weakness and numbness may last for much longer but with time recovery is usually complete.

Disc pain

This produces almost identical symptoms to facet joint pain although pain may be much more severe, but more commonly follows a direct injury to the head.

Seek medical advice. For treatment see Facet joint pain. Rarely, surgery may be required to remove a slipped disc.

Wear and tear/arthritis of the neck (osteoarthritis)

Usually pain is felt at the extremes of neck movement (bending forward, sideways or turning). The neck may click sometimes (as may a neck unaffected with arthritis).

Painkillers. Exercises to gently stretch the neck (muscles and ligaments) and a heat lamp if you have one. Ultrasound, traction and manipulation, or a collar may help. Avoid contact sports (football, wrestling, boxing, etc.) as damage can occur. Usually subsides by itself if other treatments do not work. Pain may ease but arthritis still persist.

Symptoms/Cause	Treatment

✪ Neck injury

Beware! Suspect an injury to the spinal cord if the person has been knocked out or is in severe pain. Follow the instructions in **Section Three: First Aid**.

Caused by forced movement to the neck, sometimes due to a blow to the head. There may be injury to the soft tissues only, or there may be a fracture. Spinal injury is much more common when there is a fracture, although it can be caused by injury to the ligaments alone.	Treatment of most soft tissue injuries is rest, heat, diathermy, anti-inflammatories and a collar. Worth seeking medical advice before going back to sports if the pain does not subside within a day or two. Fractures require specialist treatment in a hard collar or some sort of operative stabilization.

✪ Eye injuries

Most eye injuries are avoidable. Glasses should be of unbreakable material (polycarbonate) and in many cases contact lenses can be worn (see **Nearsightedness; Equipment**). Wear sunglasses to avoid sun or wind damage, e.g., sailing or skiing.

✪ Detached retina

Tends to occur in nearsighted people (see **Section Four: Boxing**). Seek advice before boxing if you are nearsighted. Retina (the lining at back of eye which perceives light) becomes detached from the back of the globe of the eye. The condition is not necessarily painful, but is often caused by blow to eye. Immediately after the injury or some time later, poor vision develops in eye or obscured vision in one part of eye. Loss of vision may resemble curtain being pulled across in front of part or whole of eye. If only one eye is affected it may go unnoticed until the other eye is closed.

If suspected, seek immediate medical opinion. Treatment consists of heat and laser surgery to the eye by an eye surgeon.

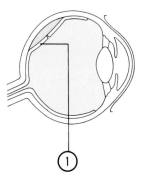

Retina (1) peels off eyeball.

Symptoms/Cause	Treatment

Sterno-costal joint strain

Can occur in people who do a lot of lifting at work. Occurs in sports involving the lifting of heavy weights, particularly push-ups or press-ups. Due to inflammation at junction of rib and cartilage at the front of the chest about three inches from the center of the breast plate. May feel lump which may be painful to touch. Made worse by twisting or breathing deeply.

Physical therapy, e.g. ultrasound, antiinflammatories, cortisone injections and rarely surgery. Not in any way a dangerous condition but may take many months to heal in some cases.

Sternoclavicular joint pain

This is the joint at the inner end of the collarbone where a bony knob can be felt. Caused by inflammation in the joint often in sports where players regularly fall on their shoulder, e.g. football. Pain is felt at the knob and may go up the side of the neck.

Treat with rest, painkillers, anti-inflammatories, sling until settled. May need ultrasound, cortisone injection. Avoid falls on the shoulder or activities that make pain worse such as lifting weights above head. Surgery rarely needed. Continue with ordinary training but avoid bench press or push-ups.

Wax rash

See **Section Four: Surfing**.

Subdeltoid bursa

Inflammation of the fluid-filled sac which lies under the deltoid muscle. This muscle raises the upper arm away from the body. Pain is felt on pulling arm from 45°- 90° from body. Caused by exercises requiring extreme power at the shoulder, such as gymnastics, weightlifting or tennis.

Treat with ice, anti-inflammatories, ultrasound and sometimes cortisone injection. Avoid exercises which aggravate the pain, e.g., press-ups, fixed cross in gymnastics, etc.

Symptoms/Cause	Treatment

Biceps tendinitis

Caused by overuse of the large biceps muscle at the front of the upper arm. More common in older people, particularly golfers. The tendon of the muscle lies within the shoulder and gets inflamed, e.g. by weightlifting or rowing. Pain is felt at the front of the shoulder while lifting and can be reproduced by bending the elbow with a weight in the hand. There is usually a tender spot at the front of the shoulder.

Rest and ice often relieve the pain. Anti-inflammatories, ultrasound and, if persistent, cortisone injection. Surgery rarely required. Train gradually, building up strength. At first, avoid lifting heavy weights with the elbow bent, and chin ups.

Bust muscle strain

Caused by strain of muscles which are attached to the chest wall at the front (pectoral muscles). Painful at certain points at the front of the chest. Pain reproduced by pressing hands inwards. Often happens in weightlifters.

Treat with rest and avoid activities which make pain worse, e.g. carrying heavy weights with the elbows away from the body. Try ice initially and painkillers. Anti-inflammatories, cortisone rarely, ultrasound and massage. Continue normal fitness routine but avoid push-ups, etc. Work gently on pectoral muscles and gradually build up the weights. Twisting exercise of upper trunk and arms may be used to stretch the muscles in recovery period and to avoid further injury.

Surfer's rub

See **Section Four: Surfing**.

Symptoms/Cause	Treatment

Impingement (subacromial bursa)

Caused by rubbing of part of the shoulder blade on the ball of the shoulder joint. This causes inflammation of the fluid-filled bag between the two bones, and pain is felt over the tip of the shoulder when the arm is vertical. Often caused by overarm activities and may be associated with painful arc.

Treat with rest and ice, anti-inflammatories, ultrasound and cortisone injection. Avoid overarm activities until the pain has settled.

Frozen shoulder

Can be caused by any injury to the shoulder although is more common after more severe types of injury particularly fractures. Due to inflammation of the lining of the joint. Joint may be swollen and hot. Pain on any movement of the shoulder and stiffness. May occur after painful arc. More common in older age groups.

Keep the shoulder moving if possible. Shortwave, ultrasound, and ice help but not heat. Anti-inflammatories, cortisone and occasionally manipulation. May take many months and up to two years to recover. However, recovery is usual in the end.

Painful arc/rotator cuff rupture

Pain in the tendons lying on top of the shoulder joint. Common in older people because blood supply to tendons is poor. Tendons may actually rupture in older people with loss of strength of shoulder. Called painful arc because pain is experienced when the arm is moved away from the body in an arc of 60''-120''. Pain made worse by activities which use an outstretched arm, such as turning a steering wheel.

Treat with rest and avoid activities which aggravate pain. Sports such as tennis, swimming and handball make matters worse. Friction and massage, ultrasound, anti-inflammatories and cortisone injections help. Rarely rupture of tendons require surgery to restore power. Calcium is sometimes deposited in the tendon and this may need removing with cortisone injection or sometimes surgery.

Symptoms/Cause	Treatment

✪ Fractured ribs

Almost always caused by a direct blow to the ribs either in a fall, a kick or similar, although severe coughing can cause it. Pain sudden and severe and breathing may be difficult initially. Cracking feeling or sound may come from the ribs as they move with breathing. May be very painful to cough. Hurts to press on ribs. Holding the chest may make breathing easier.

Painkillers and rest. Seek medical advice immediately if breathing becomes gradually more difficult after the injury; if you cough up blood (the lung may be punctured); if you have asthma or a similar chest complaint; if clicking is felt over the ribs; if there is crackling in the chest wall (air has escaped – surgical emphysema); or if there is obvious deformity of the chest. Occasionally the cavity of the chest may need to be drained if the lung has been punctured. Surgery is almost never necessary. Strapping is useless.

✪ Fractured collarbone

Caused by direct blow to collarbone or by blow to the shoulder, e.g., in judo, football or motorcycling. Pain is felt over the bone itself and the ends of the bone may be clearly visible under the skin. The fracture may move. Injuries to the underlying structures such as blood vessels and lung are rare.

Treat initially with a sling. Seek medical advice to check for other injury. Sling usually required for a week or so to hold bones in place and relieve pain. Almost always heals within three weeks although may be six weeks before safe to play football etc. Surgery rarely required. Train by using leg exercises for fitness, and keep hand and arm moving. Pendulum exercises for early movement.

Symptoms / Cause	Treatment

✪ Shoulder dislocation

Caused by blow to shoulder often in contact sport such as football or judo. May also be caused by forcing arm outwards and away from the body. The shoulder is very painful at the time, looks square and cannot be moved outwards from the body. Rarely, nerves around shoulder can be damaged and delay recovery, but complete recovery is usual.

The joint needs to be reduced (put back into the socket) as soon as possible by someone who knows what to do, otherwise, the act of reduction may complicate things by causing a fracture. It can even be difficult to do this in the hospital under anesthetic. Sling is usually required for three to six weeks. Do not take sling off too early as this may further stretch the ligaments making recurrent dislocation more likely (see below). Once sling is discarded avoid full movement of the shoulder in throwing position for first few weeks and build up strength gradually.

✪ Recurrent dislocation

Four in ten people who dislocate their shoulder sustain another dislocation (hence recurrent). This is common in those who play contact sports. It rarely does any permanent damage to the joint but can be a real nuisance and painful. The shoulder may be easy to relocate using Kocher's maneuver. However, do not try to force the shoulder back as this can cause further injury – seek medical advice. Sling is usually only necessary for a few days until comfortable.

Early return to sports is possible. Recurrent dislocation may need operation to stabilize the shoulder if it really becomes a nuisance. This means about five days in the hospital, six weeks in a sling and probably another six weeks before a return to sports. Most surgeons recommend that contact sports such as football are avoided after surgery as dislocation may recur.

Symptoms/Cause	Treatment

✪ Shoulder separation
(acromio-clavicular joint separation)

Caused by direct blow to shoulder, e.g., falling onto shoulder from motorbike, bike, judo, etc. Pain and swelling at end of collarbone. End of collarbone may be swollen and end of bone may be seen to be out of position.

Sling as first aid measure. Can usually be discarded after few days. Often permanent lump over the end of the collarbone, but usually no long-term symptoms. Surgery probably only needed in those who work with arms above head. Many football players have had this injury to both shoulders and continue playing.

✪ Torn biceps tendon/Popeye arm

Called Popeye arm because the biceps muscle (at the front of the upper arm) becomes bunched up like that of the Walt Disney figure. Occurs because the tendon of the muscle which goes through the shoulder joint becomes inflamed and breaks. Often occurs in older people with a poor blood supply. Happens in older people when they lift something heavy with their arms bent, or when a younger person sustains a sudden check when lifting a heavy weight, as in weightlifting. May occur in both arms. Often very painful for a short time, and there may be impressive bruising over the front of upper arm after a few days.

Treat with ice and rest for at least a week. Sling. Ultrasound. Exercise with gradual stretching of the muscle by straightening the elbow, and then a gradual build up of muscle strength. Does not need surgical repair. Although it looks strange, good function after a few weeks.

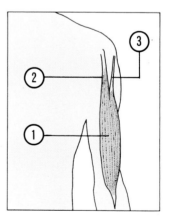

Biceps (1) means two heads. The short head (2) attaches to part of the shoulder blade, but the long head (3) runs through the shoulder joint where it can easily become ruptured.

Arm and Elbow

Symptoms/Cause	Treatment

Warning !!!!

Elbow injuries in children may be more severe than they appear. If there is any significant disability in the elbow of a child, it is best to seek medical advice. An X ray is usually done.

If the hand becomes white after the injury, pain is felt in the forearm, or if there are pins and needles in the hand, seek medical advice urgently.

Boxer's arm
See **Section Four: Boxing**.

Biceps strain

Inflammation at the point where the biceps muscle (big muscle at the front of the elbow) passes over the front of the elbow. It hurts to clench the fist or bend the elbow against resistance.

RICE initially. May need ultrasound treatment or occasionally cortisone. Rarely surgery. Usually settles in about six weeks. Avoid punching and forced bending of the elbow, push-ups or pull-ups until the pain goes. Otherwise normal training.

Pitcher's elbow
See **Section Four: Baseball/softball**.

Triceps strain

Caused by forcefully straightening the elbow, e.g. as the elbow snaps straight while throwing, or resisted straightening of the elbow when lifting weights above the head, or doing push-ups. If you try to straighten the elbow against a force, pain is felt just above the point of the elbow. Pain is caused by inflammation in the large tendon of the main muscle which straightens the elbow.

Rest is most important especially to begin with. RICE, ultrasound, massage, cortisone around the tendon. Avoid heavy weights until pain settles. Stretching the muscle at the back of the elbow by elbow bending may help.

Symptoms/Cause	Treatment

Olecranon fossa

Similar to triceps strain in that pain is felt at the back of the elbow, but the bone is to blame. Pain is felt as the elbow snaps straight, but forceful straightening of the elbow in the bent position does not hurt.

RICE, ultrasound and cortisone helps. Any exercise is okay except forcible full straightening of the elbow. When pain has gone, ease slowly back into throwing, etc, and try to avoid snapping elbow straight where possible.

Olecranon bursitis

A swelling just under the skin which may be painful. The fluid-filled sack which protects the point of the elbow gets inflamed. Caused by leaning on elbow (shooting or sailing). May become infected, with much more pain, redness in surrounding skin and fever. Almost never occurs in women.

If there are signs of infection seek medical advice. Antibiotics and drainage of pus may be necessary. If not infected, try RICE and see what happens. If swelling persists and is annoying seek medical advice. Anti-inflammatories, drainage of fluid and occasionally surgery may be needed.

Radiohumeral joint injury

Due to damage either to the ligaments around the outside of the joint or the shiny surface of the joint itself. Pain is felt over the outer side of the joint over the bony knob, as in tennis elbow. It hurts to fully twist the lower arm, fully bend or straighten it. Caused by twisting the arm downward, e.g., during a forearm tennis or badminton shot. Also caused by throwing round arm.

RICE, ultrasound, massage, anti-inflammatories and cortisone injection. Avoid activities which cause pain. Study style. See **Section Four: Badminton; Tennis; Baseball/softball**. May take much longer to settle than tennis elbow especially if the joint surfaces are affected.

Sway back elbow

See **Section Four: Gymnastics**.

Symptoms/Cause	Treatment

Tennis elbow

The muscle on top of the forearm is attached to the bone at the elbow. When this attachment becomes inflamed, it hurts to bend the wrist upward against a force, or to stretch the muscles by straightening the elbow and bending the wrist downward. Pain is felt over the bony point at the side of the elbow. There may be swelling. Caused by gripping while the elbow is bent thus affecting not just tennis players, but badminton players, canoers or rowers. Repeated throwing can cause it as can simply heavy lifting, using a screwdriver, or even typing!

RICE, painkillers, anti-inflammatories, cortisone injection, ultrasound and massage. Occasionally an operation is needed to release the inflamed area of tendons. Once pain has gone, work on stretching and building up muscle with wrist curls. Avoid lifting heavy things with the palm downward. Particularly painful hitting a backhand, therefore, an improvement in technique of this stroke is very important. (See **Section Four: Tennis.**)

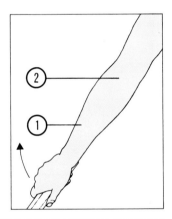

Forearm muscles (1) attach to bone at elbow (2) and it is at this point that pain from tennis elbow is felt.

Golfer's/javelin thrower's elbow

Inflammation at the site where the muscles attach onto the bone on the inner side of the elbow. Caused by recurrent stretching and strain on the muscle. Pain is felt on forced bending of the elbow or stretching of the elbow and the wrist. The bony knob on the inner side of the elbow hurts.

Stretch forearm muscles gently (the exercise will reproduce the symptoms in the early stages), RICE, anti-inflammatories, ultrasound, cortisone, very rarely surgery to release the tendon. May continue for some months. **Note: in children this may be a more severe injury – beware!**

Symptoms/Cause	Treatment

Ulnar neuritis/funny bone

Caused by repeated injury to the funny bone (ulnar nerve) which lies behind the inner side of the elbow. Pain is felt in the groove on the inner side of the elbow just behind the bony knob. May cause pins and needles or tingling in the little and ring fingers, and occasionally weakness. May be more obvious at night. Tapping the nerve may reproduce symptoms.

Avoid pressure on the nerve and activities which make condition worse. Be careful in day to day activities, such as driving with elbow on support which presses on nerve. If persistent or weakness starts, seek medical advice. Anti-inflammatories, ultrasound or cortisone. Surgical release or repositioning of the nerve may be necessary. No limitations on sports otherwise.

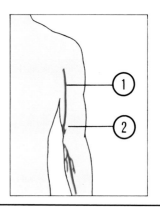

Ulnar nerve (1) runs down arm to hand. It is vulnerable to injury at elbow (2) where it runs over bone just below surface of skin.

Pronator teres syndrome

Inflammation in one of the muscles of the forearm (pronator teres). Caused by strain of muscle particularly in top-spin forearm shots. If it hurts the front of the forearm to forcibly turn the palm downward, this is the probable cause.

RICE, stretch muscle by pulling the wrist and fingers backwards and work on exercises to improve forearm strength (e.g. rotating bar with string attached and weight attached to string – rotate the bar to lift the weight upwards). Anti-inflammatories, ultrasound, cortisone, back to sports once settled.

Little league elbow/pitcher's elbow
See **Section Four: Baseball/softball**.

Wrist and Hand

Symptoms/Cause	Treatment

Shot putter's finger
See **Section Four: Athletics and field events**.

Squash player's finger
See **Section Four: Squash/racquetball**.

Lumps/ganglion

Caused by damage to the joint lining and surrounding tissues. May follow sprained ligaments of wrist. Lumps develop around wrist or at base of fingers and may get larger and smaller. They are really cysts full of joint fluid. Occur more commonly in women.

Leave alone unless troublesome or unsightly. Can be injected with cortisone, or may need operation to remove them, although 10% recur after surgery. No need to stop training.

Carpal tunnel syndrome

Numbness occurs in thumb and first three fingers. Often wakes person up at night with pain and numbness in hand and arm. Pressure over front of wrist causes pain. Often caused by repeated injury to front of wrist. Also in pregnancy and some diseases.

Rest, elevate in sling, anti-inflammatories, splint, cortisone injection, may need operation to release the nerve at the wrist particularly if troublesome or if weakness occurs in hand muscles, or numbness is persistent.

Ulnar nerve pain

May be caused by ulnar compression at elbow (see **Ulnar neuritis/funny bone**). May also be caused by pressure on the same nerve as it crosses in the palm of the hand. Again caused by pressure on the nerve, e.g., from bicycle handlebars. Causes numbness in ring and little fingers and pain at night.

Avoid pressure over nerve. RICE, anti-inflammatories, cortisone injection, very rarely release of nerve in palm.

Symptoms/Cause	Treatment

Tenosynovitis of the wrist

Inflammation of the tendons on outer side of wrist. Hurts to grip and stretch wrist to the side. Tender in one spot. Common in paddlers, rowers, and anyone who does sports gripping and rolling wrist. Also common in the general population unrelated to sports. The tendons run through a very tight canal and they get crushed.

RICE, anti-inflammatories, ultrasound, massage, cortisone injection may all help. Sometimes the only way to relieve pain is to surgically release the tendons.

Handstander's wrist

Pain felt over the back of the wrist when the wrist is turned backward. Caused by tightness in the ligaments of the wrist.

Gradually work on flexibility of the wrist. Get into a habit of gently pushing wrist backwards to improve the range of movement. Shortwave diathermy may help.

Sprained wrist

Caused by wrist being sprained by sudden movement beyond normal range. Ligaments around wrist are stretched. Wrist is swollen and hurts to move. Most painful at extremes of movement.

Strapping, RICE, rest, gradually increase activity over next six weeks. Worth protecting wrist with strapping or a splint during activity to start with. Sometimes needs professional-type splint and occasionally plaster cast for a week or two. Anti-inflammatories and ultrasound helpful.

✪ Blisters

Common sense should tell you how to avoid these. Caused by fluid building up between the layers of the skin – nature's method of protection.

If unburst and not likely to burst, leave them alone if you can resist the temptation. If they burst, leave the dead skin overlying, and keep the hand clean and dry. Watch for signs of infection. Protect the hand until the skin is hard enough to withstand pressure.

Symptoms/Cause	Treatment

✪ Finger split

Split in the skin of the hand usually in racquet sports, hockey or golf.

Adjust grip, wear a glove, cut nails back if they are the cause of the problem, tape hand before playing.

✪ Thumb sprain

The ligament on the inner side of the thumb is sprained or ruptured when the thumb is pulled outward as in skiing. The thumb swells and is painful, particularly on backward bend. There may be unusual movement at the joint suggesting rupture rather than sprain. There is usually bruising after a day or two.

Seek medical advice early because a complete rupture requires surgical repair of the ligament and ignoring the injury may lead to long-term disability. RICE very important to reduce swelling and pain. Do not put strapping on too soon as this may compress the thumb causing damage. Once swelling settles, strap. (See **Section Three: Treatments**.) If there is undue movement at the joint there may be a complete rupture of the ligament or even a fracture. Use strapping for four to six weeks. Splinting or plaster cast may be required for an injury of intermediate severity.

✪ Mallet finger

Caused by a blow to the tip of the finger, while miscatching a baseball. The finger is painful, bruised and swollen at the end joint, and the tip of the finger tends to sag.

Splint the finger straight until you can seek medical advice. Usual treatment is a mallet splint for four to six weeks, or occasionally longer. There may be a fracture which could need other treatment. Training can continue in the splint but be careful to keep finger dry underneath. Ask advice about removing splint (finger should be kept straight at all times).

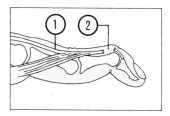

Extensor tendon (1)
Rupture (2)

Symptoms/Cause	Treatment

✪ Dislocated finger

Usually caused by a blow to the front of the finger, e.g., catching a football, basketball or baseball. The finger immediately looks deformed because the bones at one of the joints are dislocated. Initially very painful.

An attempt can be made to put the joint back by simply pulling sharply on the end of the finger. If it will not go back into joint, seek medical advice. May be associated with a fracture which needs more complicated treatment, and it may be easy to put back into joint by freezing the finger with local anaesthetic.

✪ Stress fracture of radius

See **Section Four: Gymnastics**.

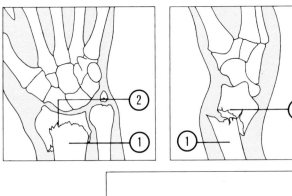

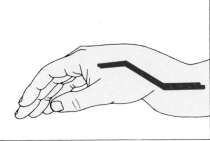

When the radius (1) fractures (2) it displaces giving rise to the typical dinner fork deformity (3).

Symptoms/Cause	Treatment

✪ Fractured radius

Break of one of the bones in the forearm which makes up part of the wrist joint (sometimes called Colles' fracture). Occurs in fall on outstretched wrist, e.g. ice skating or roller skating. Common in almost all sports. Pain at the wrist with swelling and bruising after a few hours. May be obvious deformity (dinner fork) – suggests a more severe fracture. Pain on all movements of the wrist. Often difficult to distinguish from sprained wrist (see above).

Seek medical advice. Not urgent unless very swollen, or white or numb in hand. Often simply treated in plaster cast for three weeks. Takes another three weeks to return to pre-injury sport. A more severe fracture with deformity, may need anesthetic to pull arm straight or even operation. Make sure you keep fingers, elbow and shoulder moving while in the plaster cast. Out of cast, gently push wrist backward and forward. Wrist may be swollen for many weeks after cast removed.

✪ Fractured scaphoid

Very similar mechanism of injury to radius fracture caused by a fall on outstretched hand. Pain felt in snuff box depression on outer side of wrist. May be swollen although not always. Hurts to move it. Pushing wrist backward especially painful.

If in doubt seek medical advice. Fracture not always seen on first X ray and you may be put in plaster cast for suspected fracture and X rayed again in two weeks. If fractured, expect at least six weeks in plaster as fracture is often slow to heal. Rarely needs operation. While in cast work on finger, elbow and shoulder movement. Work on other fitness, such as legs. Out of plaster gently work on moving wrist backward and forward and gripping to prevent long-term stiffness.

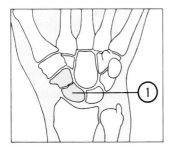

Scaphoid (1) at base of thumb.

Back

More time is lost from work in Europe and America through back injuries than from any other cause. Many, but not all, are minor and can be avoided if attention is paid to the back in daily life and in training. If you are doing a lot of lifting at work or heavy weight training, keep your back as vertical and as straight as you possibly can and use you legs to take the force of the lift. When training, work on back and abdominal muscles, particularly if you are doing a sport such as rowing or weightlifting which is known to cause back trouble. Keep your back supple – swimming and aerobics are good exercise for this, or simply do the exercises in **Section One: Getting Fit**. Keep your stomach muscles (abdominals) in good condition – these muscles take one-third of the strain when lifting heavy weights.

Training with a back problem may be difficult if not impossible. Avoid anything that hurts. Use exercises that support your back: the bench press for arms, leg press for legs. Do not use free weights. Sudden back pain may make you drop a weight and cause a worse injury. Use lighter weights than normal and do more repetitions.

Swimming is excellent exercise for fitness and for general exercise, although it is not great for building up muscle strength.

Basically you are going to have to compromise if you have a back problem. Pushing yourself too hard may only make your injury worse. Some back pain may comes from a problem in the neck. See **Head and Neck**.

Symptoms/Cause	Treatment

Ligament strain

Mechanical back problem caused largely by poor posture. Typically the pain is bad first thing in the morning and improves as the day goes on. Sitting in one position for any length of time makes it worse and it is relieved by movement. This is probably one of the most common causes of pain in the back. May occur during pregnancy due to increased body weight and laxity of the ligaments.

Try to improve your back position throughout the day. Do not sit for long periods and try to get a decent chair if you are sitting all day at work. Painkillers, anti-inflammatories, ultrasound, massage, general back exercises (see above).

Symptoms/Cause	Treatment

Bowler's back

Caused by the twisting action of bowling. It does not only affect bowlers. Typically the sharp pain comes on suddenly with the twisting movement. Due to poor alignment of the small joints in between the bones in the back (facet joints). It hurts to twist to one side or touch your toes. May be one painful spot in the back.

Rest initially. Self manipulation may work. Twist your back and you may feel a sudden click as correction occurs. If not, anti-inflammatories. Seek medical advice for manipulation.

Upper back pain

Pain felt twisting or coughing. Due to poor alignment of the facet joints in the upper back (similar to bowler's back). Occurs often in sports where the back is twisting while taking weight, as in rowing. Bending to side does not usually cause pain. There may be a painful spot just to the side of midline of back.

Rest usually settles pain within a few days. Avoid activities that hurt and avoid weightlifting until it settles. Do not lift while twisting. Anti-inflammatories, manipulation, continue with general fitness training, running, bicycling and swimming.

Gymnast's back

Common in youngsters. Caused by back arch exercise. The spine is arched back on itself and the bones in the back rub on each other causing pain. Too slow a trailing leg or too fast a leading leg causes stretching of the ligaments and muscles of the back. Pain felt in middle of back, worse when arching backwards.

Rest. Try other training techniques. Pay attention to technique (do not push youngster too fast). Improve shoulder mobility and try to achieve arch over the whole area of the back rather than over one spot. Try leading with the other leg and enlarge size of circle.

Pelvis and hip

Symptoms/Cause	Treatment

Shoulder-blade rub

Caused by rubbing of the underside of the shoulder-blade on the ribs. Grating may actually be felt. Movement of arm and shoulder hurts but back is pain-free.

Rest. Avoid exercises that hurt. Anti-inflammatories, ultrasound, cortisone injection to tender spot. Keep shoulders square during day and sports.

✪ Coccygitis (coccydynia)

Caused by fall on tailbone either once or repeatedly, or by doing exercises such as sit-ups on a hard floor. Pain at base of spine, often worse on moving the back. Can be associated with a fracture. Often painful to sit especially on soft chair.

Ice early, painkillers, antiinflammatories, ultrasound and shortwave, cortisone injection. Time often heals, and surgery rarely needed. Pain may persist for some time.

✪ Blow to flank

The kidneys lie under the flank and can be damaged particularly by something like a kick.

Rest, ice, painkillers, pain should settle within a few hours. If it does not, or if there is blood or any discoloration of the urine at any stage, seek immediate medical attention.

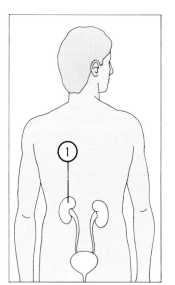

Damage to kidney (1) from a blow to the flank may cause bleeding which results in discoloration of the urine.

Symptoms/Cause	Treatment

Soccer player's groin
(osteitis pubis symphysis)

Inflammation at the point where the two sides of the pelvis join at the front. There is a ligament here (the symphysis) which becomes loose. Caused by side-stepping, (backing off from other player or hurdling) which strains this ligament. May be painful to touch at front of pelvis. Pain on sprinting or especially kicking. Due to overloading of one leg compared with other. Much more common in pregnancy. Also affects basketball and handball players.

Often takes long time to settle. Rest for at least six weeks. Gradual stretching exercises to begin with. Work on exercises to improve hamstrings, achilles' and take quads exercises very slowly.

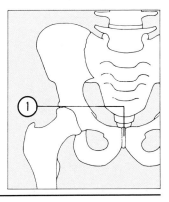

Ligament of the pubic symphysis (1).

High knee hip pain

Inflammation in the fluid-filled sac beside one of the strong muscles which bends the hip at the front. Occurs in sports where the player is bent forward (hurdles, speed skating, sprinting). Pain is felt when movement of the thigh upward toward the body is blocked.

Rest, ultrasound, cortisone. Avoid sports such as sprinting or hurdling and concentrate on general training. Look at technique – try training without sprints, running without bending the body at the hip, etc.

Adductor strain

Similar to soccer player's groin, but should be differentiated. Tender right in the groin, and pain on attempting to force the leg inward. Caused by movements with the feet pointing outward, such as side stepping, running uphill, etc.

RICE, painkillers, anti-inflammatories, massage, ultrasound, cortisone injection. Stretching exercises for the adductor muscle important in recovery period (injury caused by tension in the muscle), and also to prevent reinjury.

Symptoms/Cause	Treatment

Trochanteric bursa

Fluid-filled protective sac over the side of the hip on the bony knob gets inflamed because of direct blow, or because of unusual training regime, eg more strenuous than usual. Wiggling hips makes pain worse, and clicking may be felt over the bone.

Avoid clicking. Rest, ice, anti-inflammatories, ultrasound, cortisone injection. Train as usual but avoid pain. Surgery virtually never necessary.

Arthritis/hip joint pain

Due either to a pre-existing problem, where there is arthritis in the joint (rare before the age of 50, but can come on much earlier), or to sudden injury where there is twisting of the joint leading to a simple sprain. If arthritis, likely that you will have felt twinge of pain before in past. Either way, pain is felt in groin, particularly turning hip joint in and out. Often tender in groin. May resemble soccer player's groin but pain more to the side.

If strain, treat with rest, anti-inflammatories, ultrasound and gentle exercise. Gets better in two to three weeks. If not, then may be mild arthritis – seek medical advice. Treat with physical therapy or pool work. Surgery only usually required in severe cases. Reduce stride and avoid twisting on hip (as in golf). Work on general fitness routine such as swimming (but avoid breaststroke kick).

✪ Avulsion fracture

Caused by sudden contraction of the muscles that bend the hip at the front. Piece of bone is pulled off particularly in youngsters. Pain is felt just above the hip joint and there may be swelling and bruising as well as pain in this area.

RICE. May need six to eight weeks off sports. Almost always heals completely, but work on other muscle groups during recovery period (e.g., hamstrings, achilles' tendon muscle, and quads) but at first protect the muscles that bend the hips and work on stretching exercises.

Symptoms/Cause	Treatment

✪ Hernia (rupture)
See **Section Four: Weightlifting.**

✪ Blow to genitals (men)

Usually simply bruising to the soft tissues around the testicles, although bruising in the testicle itself can be dangerous. The other danger is damage to the pipe which carries urine (urethra).

Keep testicles cool and support in well-fitting underpants or special support. If testicles are very swollen or very painful seek medical advice. If urine is discolored or if it stings to pass urine, seek medical advice. Waterskiiers should protect this area by wearing a well-fitting wetsuit especially if inexperienced because water can be pushed in this direction at great speed during a fall.

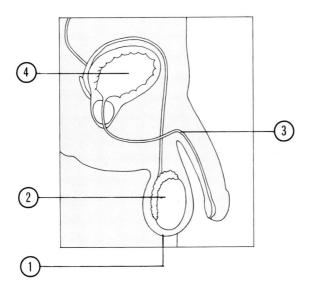

A blow to the genitals may simply bruise the scrotum (1), but the testicles (2) can be damaged. An equally serious injury is damage to the urethra (3) which drains urine from the bladder (4).

Thigh

One of the most commonly injured areas of the body in track and field events as well as in the popular sports such as football and basketball. There are many reasons for this. The muscles and tendons in the thigh are subjected to very high and sudden forces, and many sportsmen and women compete with poor training. The majority of these injuries are avoidable with the correct type of stretching and strengthening exercises.

Symptoms/Cause	Treatment

Quads insertion pull

The quads muscle (the large one at the front of the thigh) attached to the upper part of the kneecap becomes inflamed. This area can be strained by hill running, squats, step-ups, etc. Pain is felt when the upper end of kneecap is touched and it may hurt going upstairs or doing squats, etc. There may be local swelling and redness.

RICE, stretch quads muscle, avoid exercises that hurt. Massage, ultrasound and occasionally cortisone. Almost always recovers with time. Continue with usual training if comfortable.

Quads muscle pull

Inflammation of the upper part of the quads muscle, or sometimes tearing of the muscle itself with subsequent hole in the muscle. Caused by sudden blocked straightening of the knee (blocked kick), or by over-exertion of quads muscle. Painful going up stairs, cycling, lifting leg up straight while lying down, or sitting and forcibly straightening knee against resistance.

RICE, stretching, painkillers, ultrasound, sometimes surgery if there is a tear of muscle with obvious lump in thigh. Work gradually on quads in retraining with stretching exercises. Increase quads power.

Symptoms/Cause	Treatment

Hamstring sprains

Very common injuries particularly in athletes, and explosive type sports. Caused by over-stretching of the muscle and tendon due to and imbalance of power between the quads at front of leg and hamstrings at the back. More likely with insufficient warming up and stretching exercises. Not caused by a direct injury to back of thigh. Pain felt at the back of thigh, and may be painful to touch. Area may be bruised a few days after injury. Pain stretching muscle, such as touching toes.

RICE, may need to cut down sports until settled. Massage, ultrasound, stretching exercises, gradually get back into training to avoid another similar injury.

Adductor muscle strain

Hurts over inner side of thigh when touched or when leg is pulled inward toward midline against resistance. Caused by running with feet out, up hill or sprinting, for example.

RICE, massage, stretching exercises, ultrasound, strapping. Work on achilles' and hamstrings and gradually build up quads muscles.

✪ Quads injury

Often occurs in older or untrained person. Tear of the muscle at the front of the thigh. Usually sudden injury, as in a blocked kick in football. Swelling, bruising and tenderness over the quads muscle. May see lump of muscle appear at front of thigh when heel is lifted off ground with knee straight. May be difficult doing straight leg raise.

RICE. Seek medical advice as rupture may need repair. However, this is unusual and most manage to function normally with small tear. Gradually work on quads muscle. Takes at least six weeks for scar tissue to form at the rupture and to build up quads.

Knee

The knee is a hinge type joint and, unlike the hip which is a ball and socket type joint, it is much more vulnerable to damage during a twisting injury. Many of these injuries are avoidable. For example, in soccer or football foul play is quite likely to cause twisting or bending injuries which damage ligaments or cartilages. Similarly skiing is a potent way to injure the knee if bindings are not properly adjusted, or if you are an inexperienced skier and venture into deep snow. Good training of muscles can also avoid some of these injuries. However, when injury does occur and recovery is not quick, it is worth seeking medical advice at an early stage rather than waiting until stiffness has set in, making a subsequent return to fitness much slower.

Slow swelling/rapid swelling

Distinguish between slow swelling of the knee (over a space of 12 hours or longer) and quick swelling of the knee (30 minutes to 12 hours). Slow swelling usually means a ligament sprain, a cartilage tear, or injury to the lining of the joint, whereas sudden swelling of the knee suggests a more severe type of injury to the knee such as rupture of the ligaments or the cartilage, or a fracture. Sudden swelling usually signifies blood in the joint and this is best removed by needling the joint. Usually further tests are needed such as an arthrogram, arthroscopy (see **Section Three: Treatments**) and possibly an operation on the knee.

Osgood Schlatter's disease

A complicated name for inflammation of the bone at the upper end of the shin bone where the tendon from the kneecap is attached to the bone. The bony knob at the front bone just below the knee joint becomes enlarged and painful to touch. Kneeling and activities with the knee bent, such as climbing the stairs, are painful. Occurs in teenagers and is more common in boys, probably due to overloading of knee. Settles when growing stops.

RICE. Stop activities that make it worse and see if it heals. Ultrasound, perhaps time in plaster cast to rest. Avoid activities that load knee with knee bent: (bicycling, running uphill, rowing, etc.) May not heal until growth finishes.

Symptoms/Cause	Treatment

Housemaid's knee

May be mistaken for Osgood Schlatter's disease. Swelling of soft tissues over bony lump at front of upper part of shin bone where tendon is attached to bone. Caused by kneeling, or a single blow to the area. Usually simple inflammation, but may become infected, with inflammation of skin around lump, pain, temperature and difficulty bending knee.

RICE especially if caused by blow. Ultrasound, anti-inflammatories, draw off fluid, cortisone. If infected, seek medical advice as soon as possible. Antibiotics may be needed or even an operation. Avoid sports where there is much kneeling, or use knee pads.

Teenager's knee
(osteochondritis dissecans)

During growth, blood supply to the part of the thigh bone which makes the knee joint may be damaged, and a piece of bone may die and even detach and form a loose body inside the joint. May have pain, swelling and tenderness over inside of knee. Most common between the ages of 7 and 14.

Diagnosis only on X ray. Often treatment no more than simply waiting to see what happens. Often subsides on its own. May need physical therapy with exercises. Anti-inflammatories may help. Occasionally operation required to either remove or reattach loose piece.

Kneecap pain
(patello-femoral pain syndrome)

Again, common during growth, often affecting girls between the ages of 12 and 16. May be caused by kneecap being too loose or not lying normally on the end of the thigh bone. Possibly knee swelling, pain on kneeling behind kneecap, and pain climbing stairs or any exercise with knee bent, e.g., bicycling. May get clicking at back of kneecap.

Try rest, work on straight leg raise, e.g., put weight on ankle and lift up ankle with knee straight. Builds up part of muscle which maintains position of kneecap on thigh bone, and relieves pain. Brace, avoid activities that cause pain, rarely surgery to look into knee (arthroscopy), or to improve alignment of kneecap.

Symptoms/Cause	Treatment

Lower kneecap pain

May be confused with kneecap pain. Pain at the lower end of the knee-cap where the tendon attached to the bone. Caused by strain on the tendon: cycling, weightlifting, or triple jumper's who land on one leg.

RICE, ultrasound, massage, cortisone around tendon. May continue for a long time and only settle with prolonged layoff.

Jumper's knee (patella tendinitis)

Inflammation in tendon which attaches kneecap to shin bone (do not confuse with kneecap pain or lower kneecap pain), caused by strain on the ligament in jumping sports such as triple jump, hurdling, basketball, etc.

RICE, ultrasound, massage, anti-inflammatories, rest in plaster cast, very rarely needs operation to release tendon.

Hoffa's syndrome

Inflammation of the fatty tissue lying to either side of the patella tendon (tendon that connects kneecap to shin bone). Caused by repeated minor injury (overuse) during marathon running or similar. Sudden increase in activity or running on hills or hard surfaces may cause it.

RICE, anti-inflammatories, ultrasound, cortisone, change training activities.

Hamstring bursa (semimembranosus bursa)

Painful swelling behind knee on the inner side. May be caused by overuse of the hamstrings, such as cycling or running where the knee is bending rapidly. May be caused by arthritis in older people. Usually more obvious with the knee straight or while standing. May occur in youngsters.

RICE, avoid rapid knee bending. Ultrasound, massage, cortisone injection, rarely surgery.

Symptoms/Cause	Treatment

Baker's cyst

Lump appears at the back of the knee in the middle. More obvious after exercise, may give pulling sensation or pain. Often occurs in knee affected by arthritis. Often comes and goes.

Rest, little point in taking off fluid as this tends to come back. Diagnostic arthroscopy. Try to ignore and limit activities as necessary for pain, otherwise continue as usual.

Biceps bursa

Fluid-filled sac underneath biceps muscle in leg becomes inflamed. (Do not confuse with biceps muscle in arm.) Caused by fast repetitions of knee bending particularly with fast high heel lift, or running round corners. Tender and swollen just below knee joint on outer side.

RICE, anti-inflammatories, ultrasound, massage, cortisone. Avoid sprinting in training for a while, run in straight lines.

Fascia lata strain/iliotibial tract pain

On outer side of leg there is strong band of fibrous tissue which is important in supporting the knee (iliotibial band or fascia lata). Either the band itself or the point where it attaches onto the bony knob at the side of the knee can become inflamed. Usually caused by faulty technique, or running on an uneven road with bad leg down. The knee hurts when moved from straight to 30°.

RICE, adjust running technique, ultrasound, anti-inflammatories, cortisone injection, splint, rarely surgery.

Adductor avulsion

Tendon or muscle on inner side of knee is pulled off when knee is injured, as in bending injury. Pain felt just above bony knob on inner side.

RICE, anti-inflammatories, ultrasound, cortisone injection. May take long time to heal, so take medical advice.

Symptoms/Cause	Treatment

✪ Cartilage (meniscal) injury

One of the most common knee injuries. The cartilage (meniscus) acts as a spacer between the bones of the thigh and the shin. It protects the shiny surfaces of the joint from damage and provides stability. However, because the cartilages act as shock absorbers, their total removal increases the pressure on the joint by five times, so often a partial removal is carried out which means less of a pressure increase on the joint. Injury usually occurs twisting on a bent, weight-bearing knee. Knee swells within a few hours and may remain swollen for a few days. Knee may click, give way or even lock in one position, usually bent. Occurs because the torn piece gets caught between the surfaces of the joint. May be impossible to straighten knee (seek medical advice within 24 hours).

RICE in early stages. Keep quads muscle in good shape throughout treatment. Painkillers, arthrogram, arthroscopy **(Section Three: Treatments)**, or full operation to remove. Usually up to six weeks before sports can be started again. Try to avoid twisting to start with (run in straight lines and use a rowing machine).

Two cartilages, one on the inner side of the knee (1), the other on the outer (2), lie between the tibia (3) and the femur (4), underneath the patella (5). The anterior cruciate ligament (6) helps to stabilize the joint and may become torn, as can the cartilage (7).

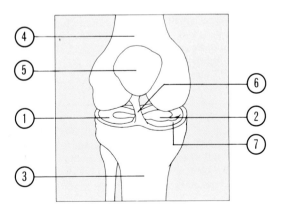

Symptoms/Cause	Treatment

✪ Dislocated kneecap

Caused either by twist on almost straight knee or by blow to knee, such as a kick. Kneecap suddenly dislocates sideways. Common in double-jointed girls. Kneecap may go out and suddenly pop back in. May need someone to push it back in. Knee often swells up within a few hours. If it swells quickly and painfully, may be associated with fracture inside joint.

RICE, seek medical advice. Usually needs splinting in plaster cast for up to four weeks on first occasion. If caused by severe blow or if fracture is present, may need operation. Dislocation may recur again and again, Important to build up quads muscle to prevent recurrence. If not, may need operation to stablilize knee joint.

✪ Fracture

Many types of fracture can occur within the knee joint. Mostly caused by direct blow to knee, although can occur with ligament injury or dislocated kneecap. More common in youngsters. Suspect if joint suddenly swells.

If suspected, seek medical advice as almost all need operation either to reattach or remove fragment.

✪ Cartilage ligament injury

The cartilage is attached to the side of the joint by a firm ligament which stops the cartilage moving around in the joint. Inflammation can be caused when these ligaments get caught in between the bones. Can be caused by running on uneven road, running with legs flailing or uphill with toes pointing outward. Catching in joint similar to torn cartilage (see above), but joint does not lock. Pain over joint line on inner side of knee.

Change training routine. Avoid running straight up hills and run up in zig-zag fashion. Do not run on uneven road, cut down mileages, make sure you are lifting knee high while running as this prevents rotation of shin bone on thigh bone which is the cause of the problem. Ultrasound, massage, anti-inflammatories, cortisone injections.

Symptoms/Cause	Treatment

✪ Medial ligament strain/rupture

Caused by forcing lower leg out sideways at the knee (valgus injury). Often occurs in skiers where there is no rotational element to injury, or in football players who get their leg caught underneath huddle. Pain felt on inner side of knee just above or below the joint. Pain occurs forcing lower leg sideways and there may be swelling and bruising over inner side of knee. If pop heard during the injury and swelling marked, may be complete rupture of the ligament rather than simple sprain.

The medial ligament (1) on the inner side and the lateral ligament (2) on the outer side help to stabilize the knee but can be torn in knee injury.

RICE, of which rest is most important. Even simple strain of ligament takes six weeks to heal. Do not try to get back to contact sports earlier than this as another injury may cause a total rupture. Support in splint, gym exercise on quads and hamstrings without weight bearing, work on arm fitness, then on to rowing machine and leg press. Ultrasound, anti-inflammatories. If injury more severe, may need period in plaster cast, either with or without knee hinge. Work on static quads while in plaster. If complete rupture, may well need surgery with recovery period of at least three months to full sports, maybe longer. Consider giving up contact sports and skiing, or using brace whenever participating because repaired ligament is weaker.

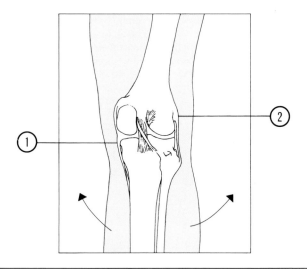

Symptoms/Cause	Treatment

✪ Lateral ligament strain/rupture

Similar to medial ligament strain, but caused by forcing lower leg inwards against knee. Pain on outside of joint just above or just below joint line. Hurts to put leg into bow-legged (varus) position. May be swollen and bruised particularly in more severe injury where there is rupture of ligament. Caused in similar way to medial ligament injury.

As for medial ligament injury. Tends to be a less severe injury than medial ligament and less frequently needs surgery.

✪ Unstable knee/cruciate ligament rupture

Called cruciate because the ligaments form the shape of a cross. They control backward and forward movement of knee and lie deep inside joint, so pain of injury may not be severe. Can be injured at the same time as other ligaments (medial and lateral), which is more severe. Usually injured by turning on knee while taking weight. May hear popping sound. Knee swells within an hour. Condition may be difficult to diagnose especially in early stages.

Seek medical advice. Strapping, splint, needle joint to remove blood, wash knee out with arthroscope (see **Section Three: Treatments**). Work on knee exercises especially quads. Most people have little or no problems once the muscle is restored, but one in three have giving way of the knee when twisting. May require surgical repair.

✪ Nerve injury

Pain and/or numbness on outer side of lower leg reproduced by pressing just below bony knob on outer side just below knee joint. Caused by blow to knee, by sitting crossed-legged for too long or by too tight a bandage or cast.

Usually recovers within two to three months if not before. Avoid pressure over nerve. Anti-inflammatories for pain. Rarely surgery if the nerve is trapped.

Lower leg

Many of these injuries are caused by overtraining, particularly running on hard surfaces for long distances. For much of the time this is really unnecessary, and fitness can be achieved just as easily by working in the gym, in the swimming pool and on a bicycle, where the leg is not subjected to the same repetitive stresses.

Symptoms/Cause	Treatment

Anterior compartment pain

Muscles at front of shin bone lie in a tight sheath. If the muscles become very enlarged by training or by prolonged exercises they do not have room to expand and this causes pain at the front of the lower leg. Particularly common in sports such as hill running because of increased strain on muscles pulling foot upward.

Change training routine, avoid step-ups, hill running, etc. RICE, painkillers, anti-inflammatories, ultrasound. If persistent may need surgery to release the muscle.

Shin splints

Caused by long distance running on hard surfaces. Scarring in the area at the front of the shin bone where the muscles attach onto the bone. Painful to touch just to the outer side of the bony ridge at the front of the shin. May resemble stress fracture though pain more diffuse.

Cut down training routine, may take many weeks to heal. Gradually build up again. RICE, especially rest, anti-inflammatories initially, ultrasound, cortisone injection, surgery. Work on exercises for achilles' strengthening.

Stress fracture

Caused by repeated minor stress to the shin bone, rather like metal fatigue. The bone does not get a chance to repair itself. Caused by running long distances on hard surfaces. Pain is felt on front of shin between ankle and knee. X ray confirms diagnosis.

Rest for six weeks often cures condition. Anti-inflammatories, ultrasound, massage. May need period of rest in plaster cast. Wear well-padded training shoes, avoid hard surface running. Use other ways of getting fit. Try shorter stride pattern and use a less high knee lift.

Symptoms/Cause	Treatment

Posterior compartment pain

Like anterior compartment pain but at back of leg. Muscle constricted in sheath due to over-development or sudden prolonged and unaccustomed exercise. Pain in the calf felt after exercise. May be tingling or numbness and pain in foot.

Ice and elevation to reduce swelling which causes problem. Painkillers. Occasionally surgery to release muscle.

Achilles' tendon pain/achilles' tendinitis

Pain in large tendon at back of ankle. Caused by repeated minor injuries in almost any sport, but particularly track and field. Pain felt to the touch over tendon and there may be a lump. May be caused by the achilles' protector at the back of some shoes (see **Section One: Protective Equipment**) which presses on the back of the tendon.

Rest and ice, may take six weeks to heal. Do not go right back to training as it will almost certainly get worse. Heel lift, massage, ultrasound, anti-inflammatories, stretching, rarely surgery. Cut achilles' protector off shoe.

Heel bone lump/calcaneal bursitis

Caused by pressing at the back of the heel from shoes. Probably caused by congenitally prominent heel bone ill-suited to modern shoes, therefore common in women who wear narrow shoes. The heel bone sac (bursa) becomes inflamed and full of fluid. Painful lump over bone at back of foot.

Train without shoes when possible. Attention to ordinary shoes, try changing training shoes or use an extra pair of socks in bigger shoe. Cover heel with tape. Anti-inflammatories, ultrasound, cortisone injections, surgery to remove lump. Try other methods of training, such as swimming, bicycling. Heel pad inside shoe may help.

Symptoms/Cause	Treatment

Outer strap muscle pain

Caused by inflammation in the tendons which pull the foot outward. May follow a sprained ankle. Pain is felt pulling the foot outward against pressure, and may be tender below outer ankle bone. There may be a clicking feeling here on moving the foot. Caused by pigeon-toed running, or a tendency to run on the outer side of the foot.

RICE, cut down training schedule, attention to technique, strapping, heel wedge to build up outer side of shoe, anti-inflammatories, ultrasound, cortisone, surgery to release tendons.

Inner strap muscle pain

Similar to outer strap muscle pain, but on the inner side of the ankle. Pain felt behind inner ankle bone, may extend into the foot. Pain on pressure, and clicking may be felt moving the foot up and down. Pain on forcing the foot inward against pressure. Tends to occur in people who run on the inside of the foot or those who are flat-footed. Sports where you roll inward on the foot, such as squash, may cause this.

Improve muscle tone in foot by exercises to improve arches. Stand on tiptoe, try to pick up objects with toes. Inner sole arch support, heel wedge on inner side of shoe. Anti-inflammatories, ultrasound, massage, cortisone injections, surgical release of tendons. Alter training schedule.

✪ Calf muscle strain

More common in older individuals. Tearing within muscle on sudden stretching or unaccustomed exercise, e.g., landing awkwardly on tiptoe. May feel as if someone has kicked you from behind. Pain felt in large muscle at back of calf, painful or weak on tiptoe, swelling and bruising, sometimes further down leg a few days later. Do not confuse with achilles' tendon rupture.

RICE, painkillers, anti-inflammatories for a few days. May take five to six weeks to heal. Gentle stretching exercises, work on other muscles in gym not taking weight on calf muscle. Ultrasound, massage.

Symptoms/Cause	Treatment

✪ Ruptured achilles' tendon

Must be differentiated from calf muscle strain. May also feel as if you have been kicked from behind, but pain, swelling and bruising is at the lower end of the calf muscle or more commonly in the tendon itself. You may be able to feel a gap in the tendon where it is broken. Impossible to stand on tiptoe on one leg. Squeezing calf when kneeling on chair fails to cause the foot to point away.

Avoid by stretching exercises before sports. Warm up properly. After injury, rest, ice and elevation. Seek medical advice as soon as possible because surgery is nearly always needed immediately. Plaster for six weeks. Heel lift after, and stretching exercises. Re-rupture can occur and is more common in cases where no operation is performed. Consider changing sport if older age group. Very gradual achilles' strengthening exercises.

✪ Fracture of shinbone

Quite common in contact sports, football, basketball. Direct blow to shin. **Note: not stress fracture**. Diagnosis usually obvious.

Do not take weight on leg. Elevate, splint, seek medical advice immediately. Usually treated in plaster cast, but may need operation. Takes minimum of three months to heal and sometimes much longer. Work on knee movement, and thigh muscles. Move calf muscles as much as allowed in cast. Out of plaster work on ankle movement and build up muscle strength in gym, not taking weight initially through leg. Take medical advice about what you can and cannot do. Usually lose season from sport, e.g., football or skiing.

Ankle

The ankle takes much of the force of twisting injuries together with the knee. When the ankle is well supported, as in a ski boot, these forces are transmitted to the shin bone and the knee ligaments. The joints in the foot act to convert a simple inward or outward force on the foot into a twisting force, which may then damage the ligaments or bones around the ankle. It is often difficult to tell if you have damaged something serious, so if in doubt, seek medical advice.

Symptoms/Cause	Treatment
### Shoe pain	
Rubbing, blisters and ulcers caused by the plastic shoe decorations put on shoes by manufacturers, which do not expand with rest of shoe.	Plaster or tape over area. Cut junction of plastic and sole of shoe. Change shoes. Keep rubbed area clean and dry to avoid infection.
### Flat foot pain	
Flat foot running causes pain over the inner strap muscles (see section on lower leg and calf injuries), and sometimes pain from rubbing over the outer ankle bones. Hurts to lift foot up and outward.	Buy good supportive shoes. Strap (see page 120). Inner arch support on inner side of foot. Work on small muscles of foot to improve arch by curling toes down and holding an object, and fanning toes outward.
### Stress fracture of fibula	
Fibula is a thin bone on the outer side of the ankle joint. Pain is felt about six inches from the sole of the foot on the outer side of the lower leg. Caused by running bow-legged or pigeon-toed, although it may occur in anyone who does a lot of running, particularly on hard surfaces over long distances. Tender to press on the area and may be swollen.	RICE. May take six weeks to recover. Maintain fitness with swimming and bicycling which does not stress bone in the same way. Anti-inflammatories, strapping, plaster cast sometimes if it does not settle.

Symptoms/Cause	Treatment

Soccer player's ankle

Painful, stiff ankle. Called soccer player's ankle because it is due to repeated kicks around the ankle and minor ankle sprains. Scarring in the ligaments around ankle can lead to formation of new bone around the ligaments, hence the stiffness.

ICE, strapping, shin pads which protect ankle, anti-inflammatories. Continue as usual with sports.

Fosbury flop ankle

See **Section Four: Athletics and field events**.

Jumper's/dancer's heel

Caused by snapping the heel bone against the bottom of the shin bone compressing the fat pad between the bones or sometimes compressing another small bone between them. Caused by standing on points, explosive jumping or trapping ball at soccer with the toes pointing towards the ground. Pain felt to either side of achilles' tendon.

Avoid activities that worsen condition, and rest. Anti-inflammatory drugs, ultrasound, cortisone injection, rarely surgery.

Pinched heel

Pain under heel due to bruising from repeated injury or single blow to bottom of heel bone.

Keep off heel. Put special heels pads in shoes.

Young runner's heel

Also called Sever's disease. Only affects growing bone and pain is felt over back of heel. Hurts landing on heel or jumping.

RICE. Anti-inflammatories, avoid activities that make things worse, especially running. Concentrate on exercises such as swimming, bicycling, rowing. Gets better when growing finishes.

107

Symptoms/Cause	Treatment

✪ Sprained ankle

One of the most common of all injuries. Happens when the foot turns under. Pain felt over the outer side of the ankle. Tender to touch, hurts to push the foot inward. Swelling, bruising at outer side of ankle on or just below outer ankle bone. Bad bruising or swelling suggests a complete rupture of the ligament rather than a sprain. This can be confused with a fracture of the ankle, so if in doubt seek medical advice. Occasionally stiffness of ankle may persist for more than six weeks after sprain. Try exercises, manipulation of the ankle, cortisone.

RICE very important to start with or swelling increases and injury takes longer to heal. Elevate for 48 hours if possible. Strapping for ankle (see page 120). May need crutches for a few days if too painful, but if a simple sprain you should be able to walk on ankle almost immediately. Avoid tiptoes as this is an unstable position for the ankle and you may sustain another injury. Practice on ankle wobble board once no longer painful. Anti-inflammatories, ultrasound, massage. If complete rupture, doctor may suggest up to six weeks in plaster to avoid ankle instability. Continue on arm exercises, and start with non-twisting exercises to avoid another injury.

✪ Inner ankle sprain

Similar to outer ankle sprain but on other side of ankle. Less common. Occurs when the foot turns over outward. Fracture more likely than with injury on outer side.

See **Sprained ankle**.

✪ Unstable ankle

Frequent giving way of the ankle may follow a single or many ankle sprains, or a complete ankle rupture which was not treated in plaster cast at time of injury. Difficult to diagnose.

Work on muscles that pull the foot outward using ankle wobble board, and use strapping for support (see page 120). Avoid running downhill on rough ground. Plaster cast, surgical repair of ligament.

Symptoms/Cause	Treatment

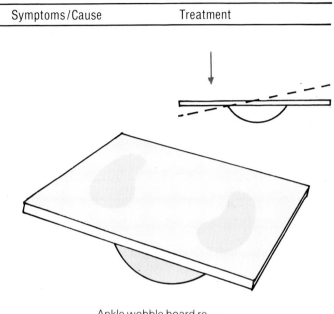

Ankle wobble board re-educates and strengthens the muscles which turn the foot from side to side thus preventing further sprains.

⭐ Broken ankle bones (fracture)

Same method of injury as for sprained ankle and inner ankle sprain. Fracture may occur on inner or outer side of the ankle bones. Ankle usually swollen with bruising which appears within a few hours, and movement of the ankle hurts. May be impossible to walk on the ankle. Often difficult to tell from sprain of ankle, so if in doubt, seek medical advice.

Some fractures treated as for ankle sprain and if so usually heals within three or four weeks. Most other fractures treated in plaster cast for three to six weeks. More severe fractures treated with operation and metalwork to hold fracture in place while it heals. Once free of plaster, work on ankle movement, ankle wobble board, achilles' tendon exercises, swimming, bicycling, then running in straight lines, not on rough ground. Finally return to sports once ankle is really stable.

Foot

Shoes are all important in preventing many of these injuries. (See **Section Two: Protective Equipment**.) Try to get the shoes that suit your sport best, and avoid buying shoes that are too heavy or do not give adequate support for your sport. Use common sense and break in shoes properly. There is no point in going right out and running 20 miles in one day if you are not used to it. Trim nails regularly and always wash feet after sport as this lessens the chance of infection. If you develop a problem such as a blister, treat it early rather than waiting for it to develop into a big problem.

Symptoms/Cause	Treatment
## March fracture	
So called because it is common in young army recruits who have to march long distances. Caused by repeated stress on the small bones in the foot. Long distance road running can cause this. Hurts to exercise and press on back of foot.	Avoid in first place by doing long distance running on soft surfaces and wearing shoes with adequate sole protection. After injury, RICE. Wear shoes with a firm sole for support for every day. Stop running until it settles completely. May need plaster cast. Sometimes very slow to heal. Stick to swimming, cycling, rowing, and similar training which does not cause repetitive loading of the foot.
## Metatarsalgia	
Pain under the ball of the foot due to damage to the fat pad underneath the bones. May be simple bruising or more permanent inflammation. Pain felt on pressing the area.	If due to single bruising type injury, RICE usually helps it quickly. Wear well-padded shoes, run on soft surfaces. Cut a pad out and stick on inner sole so that it lies just behind the painful bones, thus taking some of pressure off the bones. Physical therapy with intrinsic muscle exercises (exercises for the small muscles in the foot). Rarely surgery.

Symptoms/Cause	Treatment

Navicular pain

Very similar to march fracture, but different bone (the one on inner side of foot just beyond ankle joint).Caused by repetitive loading of the bone in running, etc. Hurts to take weight on foot and press on bone.

See **March fracture.**

Sesamoid pain

Sesamoid is a tiny bone within tendon to big toe on sole of foot. Pain felt on ball of foot under big toe at base. Caused by landing heavily on ball of foot, as in squash, high jump, running on hard surfaces. May even get fracture of bone or arthritis in tiny joint in bone.

RICE, anti-inflammatories, train without running, e.g., swim, row, cycle, get back to sport in well-padded shoe on soft surfaces. Ultrasound, cortisone, plaster cast, very rarely surgery.

Heel spur/plantar fasciitis/calcaneal spur/triple jumper's heel

Due to stretching of very strong spring ligament on sole of foot. Attachment of ligament to heel bone (calcaneus) becomes inflamed by repeated damage during jumping (hence name), or other sports such as squash, road running, etc. Common in overweight people. May be spur at front of heel bone, visible on X ray. Pain felt on inner side of sole of foot at front of heel bone.

Rest, ice, elevate, heel shock-absorber in shoe. Cut out pad with hole under tender area and place in shoe. Arch support. Anti-inflammatories, cortisone, training on bike, swimming, rowing. Surgery almost never required.

Symptoms/Cause	Treatment

Morton's neuroma

Often confused with metatarsalgia. Nerve between the metatarsal bones gets squashed and forms neuroma (lump on nerve). Pain felt between bones in ball of foot. Neuroma may be felt clicking in and out. May be tingling or numbness in adjacent toes.

Pad as for metarsalgia. Ultrasound, cortisone, surgery to remove neuroma (will make adjacent toes numb). Continue training as usual but avoid tight shoes.

High arch pain

May be due to high arched foot. Foot only painful wearing shoe. May be obvious signs of rubbing.

Buy shoes that fit properly. Stretch shoes. Pad back of foot. Check arch support is not causing problem by pushing foot upwards.

Callouses on toes

Caused by abnormal rubbing. Can occur on any pressure points on the foot, particularly over the back of the toes due to shoes being too short and toes cramped, or due to shoes being too tight at the sides.

Common sense about shoes. If persistent problem, may need to see podiatrist who can trim redundant dead skin.

Surfer's foot

See **Section Four: Surfing**.

Strained front of ankle joint

Similar to soccer player's ankle. Sprain of the ligaments at the front of the ankle. May be caused by blocking kick while kicking with back of foot, or falling with foot caught behind leg. Pain felt at front of ankle joint on pressure and hurts to push foot downward.

RICE. Anti-inflammatories, strapping. Ultrasound, massage.

Symptoms/Cause	Treatment

Arthritis

More common in older age group. May occur in any of joints in foot, but most common in joints at back of foot and in ankle joint. Pain felt on exercise but also at rest and at night. All movements painful but most painful at extremes. May be swelling and tenderness around affected joints.

Rest, elevation, anti-inflammatories, exercises to improve muscle power, massage, ultrasound, diathermy. Do not over-exercise.

Skater's heel
See **Section Four: Skating**.

Ingrown toenail

A nuisance particularly for teenage boys. Causes infection, pain and inflammation in the corner of the nail, thought to be caused by not cutting nail properly – should be cut straight across rather than in curve to corner of nail. Made worse by dirty, sweaty feet.

Cut nail correctly. Try to cut off piece of sharp nail which is causing problem. If persistent, seek medical advice. Antibiotics, operation to remove nail or to prevent part or all of nail growing again.

Rigid toe/hallux rigidus

Caused by arthritis in the big toe joint. This type of arthritis does not spread elsewhere. Hurts to push toe backwards. Joint is stiff and may be enlarged and tender.

Rest, wear shoes with firm sole to support toe. Gentle movement of joint, massage, anti-inflammatories, cortisone, possibly surgery although most operations make push off worse and may make sports more difficult.

Symptoms/Cause	Treatment

✪ Black nail/runner's toe/turf toe

Caused by damage to nail bed. May be caused by a direct blow to the nail, e.g. someone treading on toe. Painful bruise occurs under toenail and nail may eventually drop off. May be caused by continuous injury to nail, e.g., by shoes being too short. May be very painful if bruise occurs quickly.

Elevation, ice. Try changing shoes if too tight.

✪ Fractures

Usually caused by direct blow to foot (someone standing on foot or fall from height). Many types of fractures may result. Foot is swollen, painful, bruised.

Elevation, ice, seek medical advice. May need crutches, plaster cast but rarely surgery.

✪ Blisters

Usually caused by rubbing from either poorly fitting shoes or unaccustomed activity, such as marathon running. Occurs over points of pressure.

Avoid by attention to shoes and common sense. If blisters occur, burst blister and leave dead skin overlying tender new skin to protect. Keep feet clean to avoid infection and protect area against further pressure, for instance by taping area for sports. If signs of infection (swelling, redness, tenderness and heat) seek medical attention.

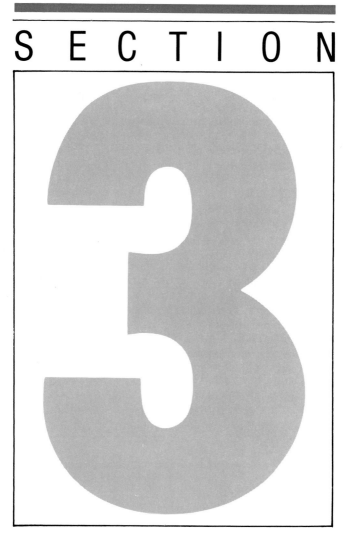

FIRST AID
TREATMENTS

Treatments

First Aid

Loss of consciousness, usually due to a head injury, is a common problem in sports and, although in most cases the player recovers completely, it is ALWAYS a potentially life-threatening situation and should be treated very seriously. It is advisable for all trainers, coaches or players involved regularly in sports to take a proper First Aid course because the use of artificial respiration and heart massage can save a life but to be effective must be carried out IMMEDIATELY, and cannot wait even a few minutes for professional help to arrive. The most common cause of death in an unconscious person is an obstruction of the airway and in most cases correct First Aid techniques can prevent this.

If the player is breathing normally, he or she may be put into the recovery position which ensures that the mouth and nose remain clear if the player vomits. If there has obviously been a serious neck injury AND the person is still breathing normally, it is not advisable to move the head at all but watch the person's breathing ALL THE TIME while you wait for professional help to arrive.

If the player is not breathing or is breathing with difficulty (gargling, gasping or breathing irregularly), start resuscitation.

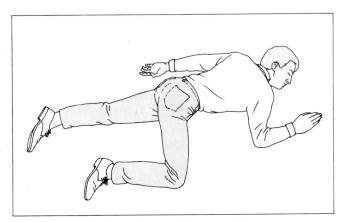

The Recovery Position

Kneel and gently turn the person onto his or her side. Draw one arm and one leg up to make a right angle with the body, and place the underneath arm backwards. Turn the head to one side.

Cardiopulmonary resuscitation

This is not difficult but is potentially very hazardous if you do not know exactly what to do. You need to practice the procedure, and the only way to do this is on a dummy during a First Aid course. NEVER try it on a healthy person.

ABC of resuscitation is **Airway, Breathing, Circulation.**

Airway

Lie the player on the back, lift the chin up, remove any obstruction in the mouth such as dentures, mouth shield, vomit, blood or broken teeth as far down as you can reach. This may be enough to start the person breathing again. If not start mouth to mouth resuscitation.

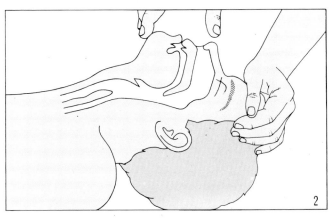

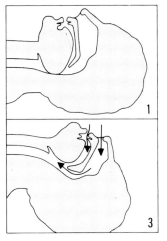

Clearing the Airway

The tongue of an unconscious person can fall to the back of the throat (1) and prevent the person from breathing. Raising the chin (2) lifts the tongue forwards and is often enough to free the airway (3).

Breathing
Keeping the chin up, pinch the nose and breathe out into the person's mouth at the same time as watching the chest which should expand. Take your mouth away and the person's chest falls, expelling the air while you take another breath yourself. Continue at your own breathing rate. After three or four breaths check that the person's heart is beating by feeling for a pulse at the side of their Adam's apple. If it is, continue mouth to mouth resuscitation until breathing begins or help arrives. If not, begin cardiac massage.

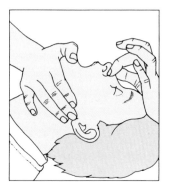 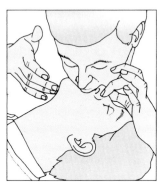

Mouth to Mouth Resuscitation
Keep the person's chin up with one hand and use the other to hold the nostrils shut. Place your lips around the mouth and make sure you have an airtight seal. As you breathe out into the person's mouth, watch to make sure the chest rises. If it does not, there is an obstruction and you must check the airways again.

The Carotid Pulse
The easiest place to feel a person's pulse is at the side of the Adam's apple where the large carotid artery runs up the neck.

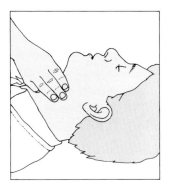

Circulation

If the heart has stopped it is possible to pump blood around the body artifically by rhythmically squeezing it with hard pushes on the breastbone. This is called external cardiac massage. Take a course and learn how to do it.

Bleeding

The sight of blood on the sports field is often alarming, but rarely serious. Nevertheless it is important to know how to deal with it.

Wherever the injury, the basic principal is the same. Lie the player down, raise the injured limb, and press firmly on the wound, ideally with a sterile dressing. Pressure will always stop bleeding and should be applied directly to the wound. It is NEVER necessary to use a tourniquet, in fact it is dangerous.

RICE

Rest, Ice, Compression, Elevation

This can be applied in most sports situations within a few minutes of injury, and the sooner the treatment is started, the more effective it is. Do not feel tempted to finish the game after an injury as this may increase your recovery time. RICE lessens inflammation by reducing swelling and bruising which occur after injury.

Rest

Stop play and rest the injured part. Splint if necessary.

Ice

Applied to the injured area. Anything cold will do: a cooled can of soda, a package of frozen peas, or crushed ice in a plastic bag but protect the skin with a towel first. Do not leave on unprotected skin for more than 15 minutes or if it becomes painful as this may cause damage. Apply every two hours for the first few hours.

Compression

After ice, bandage area firmly but not too tightly as this may cut off the circulation. Remove at two hourly intervals, apply ice and rebandage. Remove immediately if pain is severe or if limb becomes white or blue.

Elevation

Reduces swelling and throbbing pain. Put foot on stool if leg injured, or arm in high sling.

Splints

These are used for two reasons:

1. To immobilize an injured joint to rest it. There are specific polyethylene splints to fit the knee, ankle, wrist, etc., but suitable temporary splints can be made in an emergency from cardboard or padded wood.

2. To immobilize a fracture (or suspected fracture) during transport to the hospital. There are many commercially available varieties and the more sophisticated inflate around the injured limb. However, an effective splint can be made from anything suitable such as a cane. At worst, an injured leg can be strapped to the good leg and an injured arm to the body.

In either case take care that the splint is well padded and the bandages holding it are not too tight. Regularly check the circulation in the fingers or toes by making sure they are pink and warm. The limb should be more comfortable in the splint and if the pain worsens or the circulation is cut off, remove the splint.

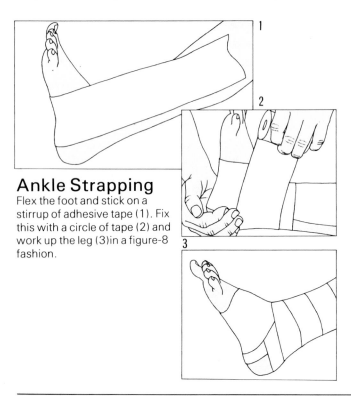

Ankle Strapping

Flex the foot and stick on a stirrup of adhesive tape (1). Fix this with a circle of tape (2) and work up the leg (3) in a figure-8 fashion.

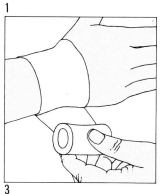

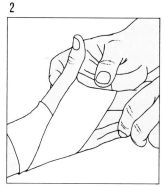

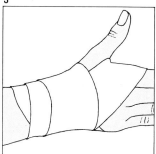

Wrist Strapping

Wrap a layer of tape around the wrist (1) then up between thumb and fingers (2) and back. Continue strapping as shown in (3).

Thumb Strapping

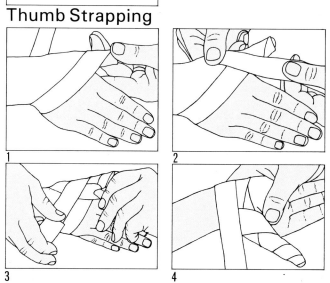

Wrap tape around tip of thumb and down across back of hand (1), around wrist (2), down towards joint and around thumb (3). Build up the layers finishing with a strap around wrist (4).

Medication

The misuse of drugs in sport is widely known and deplorable but there are some drugs such as painkillers (analgesics) which are valuable in the treatment of sports injuries.

It is worth remembering that due to the misuse of drugs in sports, drug testing at competitions is now standard and some prescribed and over-the-counter medicines used legitimately for unrelated illnesses such as diarrhea or travel sickness may ban you from competition. If in doubt, check with your doctor and the testing authorities.

Anabolic steroids are widely used for increasing muscle mass. They allow the athlete to train longer and more frequently but have not been shown to increase performance. The increase in muscle mass tends to stress the other tissues, leading to increased soft tissue injuries. There does seem to be a psychological effect from the drugs which diminishes achievement. Anabolic steroids damage the liver, suppress sperm production and raise blood pressure. They should never be used in children as this can damage growth, and should not be used in women due to the masculinizing effect of the drug, which can also cause damage to the fetus if the woman is pregnant.

Analgesics are painkillers, the most common being aspirin and acetaminophen. Aspirin also has a strong anti-inflammatory effect (see below). They are freely available and very valuable in the first few days following injury in association with RICE. If the pain persists seek medical advice rather than trying to get back to your sport by continuing to take them. Stronger analgesics are available from your doctor and may be necessary following severe injury.

Antibiotics, available on prescription only, are used for bacterial infections such as in the middle ear but have no effect on viruses such as cause the common cold and flu. Side effects include diarrhea and skin rashes.

Anti-inflammatories are drugs which reduce inflammation. They are widely used in the treatment of arthritis but can also help after injury by reducing pain and swelling. They are particularly valuable in conditions such as tenosynovitis and knee injuries. Ibuprofen is one of the most widely used but there are many others available. They all have a similiar action and share the side effect of stomach irritation.

Some people have used them before sports in anticipation of injury but this is not recommended because they dampen the body's natural protective and healing response and may do more harm than good.

Betablockers were designed for the treatment of high blood pressure but are widely used for control of anxiety and tremor especially in marksmen although they have been shown to decrease performance in athletes.

Cortisone is a steroid which occurs naturally in the body. It has a potent anti-inflammatory effect and is used in sports medicine in the form of an injection into an inflamed area such as a tennis elbow which has failed to respond to simple treatment and rest. Even though a local anesthetic is mixed with the steroid before injection, it is painful and uncomfortable for a few days afterwards before the steroid begins to have an effect. Several injections may be needed over a period of a few months although there is a limit to the amount of injections you can have in any one spot. It only

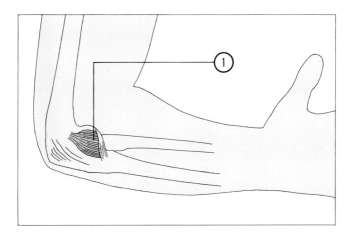

Cortisone Injection for Tennis Elbow
In tennis elbow, the pain is confined to a small area where the muscles of the forearm attach onto the bone. This makes it suitable for a single local injection (1) which reduces the inflammation.

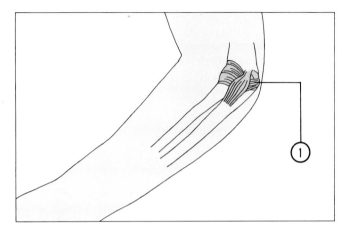

Cortisone Injection for Golfer's Elbow

In golfer's elbow, the pain is felt where the muscle attaches onto the bone on the inside of the elbow (1).

works where it is injected and does not have an effect on the rest of the body.

Liniment is a pain-relieving skin rub which acts by mildly inflaming the skin and stimulating a soothing heat. No chemicals actually pass into the body.

Painsprays are simply cold sprays which freeze the skin reducing pain temporarily.

Stimulants such as amphetamines are misused widely by athletes in an attempt to increase work output and decrease fatigue. They are, however, potentially dangerous, some are addictive and there is no place for them in the management of sports injuries.

Tetanus toxoid is a vaccine. It is given by injection and is part of the standard vaccination program of children in this country. Tetanus (lockjaw) is an extremely serious disease. You can get it from a dirty cut or scratch which may not need any form of medical attention. It is therefore essential for all athletes to have regular booster injections every five to ten years to maintain protection.

Physical therapy

The mainstay of treatment of sports injuries because it maximizes the athlete's potential to return to his or her sport quickly and safely after injury. It does this by reducing the pain and swelling of the injury at the same time as maintaining movement and muscle power while natural healing occurs.

Diapulse is a form of ultrasound (see below).

Faradism is used to artificially stimulate paralyzed or weak muscles by applying an alternating current to the limb with electrodes.

Interferential uses two different medium frequency alternating currents which are applied either side of the injured area. Three or four pads pass electrical currents through the body. The waves cross at a certain point and interact with one another in such a way that the tissue being treated heats up. It can be used for ligament sprains, capsulitis of the shoulder, tenosynovitis and low back pain. Usually up to 12 treatments are used.

Manipulation is the passive movement of a joint by the therapist to increase its range of movement and reduce pain. It is commonly used for spinal problems and is particularly valuable to unlock a locked joint of the back when the results can be dramatic. It is not a substitute for a training program which should include stretching and strengthening exercises.

Massage is one of the oldest forms of physical therapy but still has a place in the management of some sports injuries although the more modern techniques of interferential and ultrasound are taking its place. Early massage probably helps to reduce inflammation, and frictional massage is useful in the later stages of treatment for scarring and swelling.

Shortwave diathermy is similar to interferential but uses only one high frequency current to heat up the tissues. Either applied with electrodes or a coil close to the injured area which sets up a magnetic and electrical field within the tissues. The treatment should reduce inflammation, swelling and pain and increase blood supply in damaged tissues, as well as producing muscle relaxation.

Traction is the gentle stretching of the spine by a device of straps and weights applied to the neck, lower back and pelvis. This aligns the spine correctly, reduces muscle spasm and relieves pressure on the spinal nerve roots. Usually used for 15 to 30 minutes, two or three times a week for up to four weeks.

Ultrasound uses inaudible sound waves to stimulate damaged tissues, reduces pain and inflammation and is thought to promote healing. A gel is put on the skin to improve conduction and a small probe is moved gently over the injured area.

Specialist treatment

A wide variety of specialist surgical and medical techniques may be necessary for sports injuries but arthroscopy and arthrography are two of the most common.

Arthroscopy is the technique of looking into a joint with a telescope. It is carried out in a hospital under local or general anesthetic and is extremely valuable in the management of knee problems, particularly torn cartilages. It allows the surgeon to diagnose the problem accurately and, in many cases, treat it without a major operation. The advantage of this is that it is less painful and recovery is much quicker, and in some instances the procedure can be performed as outpatient surgery.

The knee is filled with water, saline or gas and two or three tiny holes are made over the front of the knee for insertion of the arthroscope and operating instruments. The surgeon can get a good view of both cartilages and the anterior cruciate ligament, as well as the shiny surfaces of the joint. If one of the cartilages are torn it can usually be cut away and pulled out through one of the small holes. In some cases the surgeon will find a problem that cannot be treated through the arthroscope and may have to proceed to a bigger operation. He or she will explain this to you before surgery.

It is surprising how quickly the knee becomes pain free after arthroscopic surgery but do not be tempted to get back to sports too soon. It may be six weeks before you are ready to return to full activity. During this recovery period, start by working hard on isometric quadriceps exercises (static quads), using ice if necessary, and then gradually build up to more active exercises such as swimming and cycling.

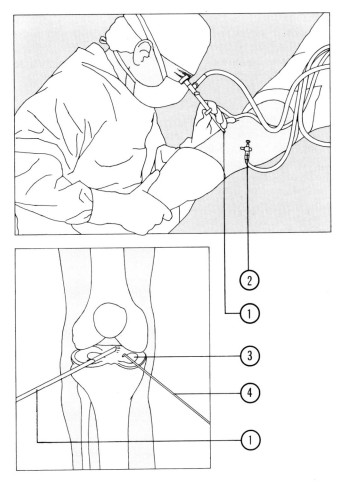

Arthroscopy

Under anesthetic the surgeon can examine the inside of the knee with an arthroscope (1) while the joint is filled with water (2). This allows accurate examination of the cartilages (3). Operations can also be carries out with instruments (4) inserted into the joint.

Avoid twisting movements of the knee or competitive sports until you are confident and the surgeon has given you the all clear. Remember you will be getting over not just the arthroscopy but also the injury which made the arthroscopy necessary.

Arthrography is a special type of X ray which is used to diagnose disorders of the cartilages, ligaments and shiny surfaces of the inside of a joint, usually the knee. These structures are made of cartilage and do not show up on conventional X rays.

Iodine-containing fluid (contrast material) and gas are injected into the joint and X rays are then taken of the knee in various positions. The internal structures now coated with the contrast material are visible on X ray and any abnormality can be seen.

This is performed as an out-patient technique under local anesthetic. It only takes an hour or two and is not particularly painful although the knee remains uncomfortable for some days afterwards, so do not have it done just before a competition or other event.

The advantage of arthrography over arthroscopy is that you do not need to be admitted to hospital, and it is relatively quick and easy. The disadvantage is that if there is an abnormality which needs surgery, this will have to be done at a later date rather than at the same time.

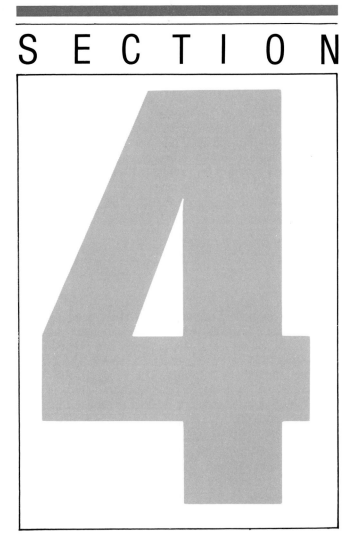

SPORTS-SPECIFIC INJURIES

Sports-Specific Injuries

This section looks at the injuries specific to particular sports disciplines and some technique changes are suggested. Conditions in bold type are explained more fully in **Section Two**, but a condition which only occurs in certain sports (such as Fosbury flop ankle) is discussed here. When treatment suggests RICE, see page 119.

Archery

All injuries can be avoided if correct technique is taught in the first place. However, **Tennis elbow** can affect the arm which holds the bow and **Biceps strain** can occur in the other arm if the drawweight is too heavy. Have your technique checked by a trainer. The string should never cause injuries so arm and chest protectors only help if a person's technique is wrong. It is better to get coaching and forget the protectors.

Athletics and field events

Some athletes strain muscles frequently, others hardly at all. People who are less supple are more prone to muscle and tendon injury than those with very lax joints. Most of the injuries from these sports affect the legs and feet but many can be avoided by wearing the correct type of shoe and using the exercises described in **Section One**.

Adductor strain and **Hamstring sprains** are some of the common injuries in this group. They are more common in athletes who take part in explosive actions such as sprinting rather than sustained activities like middle-distance running. Hamstring injuries are often caused by running perpetually in an anticlockwise direction around running tracks and can be avoided if training runs are carried out in the opposite direction.

Quads injury, Osgood Schlatter's disease and **Jumper's knee** (patella tendinitis) are quads mechanism injuries. Kicking exercises aggravate these conditions. **Soccer**

player's groin (osteitis pubis symphysis) can affect hurdlers and discus throwers. See also **Kneecap pain** (patello-femoral pain syndrome).

Fosbury flop ankle is common in high jumpers and is caused by the rotation of the lower leg on the foot during take off. The lower bone of the ankle joint is compressed against the lower end of the shin bone at the ankle joint. This damages the shiny surface of the joint and sometimes the underlying bone. It hurts to push the foot upward and outward. RICE, anti-inflammatory drugs, strapping and a change of technique to avoid re-injury are the best treatment. Try straightening your running technique. If the ankle continues to be troublesome, cortisone injections may help. Occasionally an operation on the underlying bone is needed.

Golfer's/javelin thrower's elbow is an injury to the inner side of the elbow caused by a round-arm style of throw. Considerable forces are applied to the elbow in acceleration and follow through. In an adult this results simply in inflammation of the muscle attachment (where the muscle is joined to the bone), but in children a piece of bone may be pulled off, so it is important to seek medical advice for this condition which may need surgery.

Shot putter's finger is a sprain of the first three fingers of the hand, those used in the final stages of acceleration. The pain is felt on the sides of the fingers. The best way to treat this injury is to avoid using the fingers to get the final bit of acceleration during training sessions, reserving this for competitions. Strapping may help although this may be illegal in competition. Alternatively, treatment by a physical therapist and/or ultrasound helps.

Shin splints and **Stress fracture** affect athletes who train by running long distances on hard surfaces.

Badminton

A demanding sport, so pay attention to fitness with one or two training sessions a week even if it is only going for a run. Stretching exercises are a must.

Baseball/softball

Potentially hazardous sports because they attract the relatively unfit who play on an occasional or weekend basis and people underestimate the fitness required to run, bend, turn and field the ball.

The elbow joint comes under enormous stress during a round-arm throw causing pain on the inner side, or back of joint, known as pitcher's elbow. This is caused by inflammation where the muscles are attached to the bone because these are stretched during the final act of throwing, acceleration and follow-through. Pitcher's elbow is best treated with RICE but persistent symptoms may require physiotherapy in the form of ultrasound, or anti-inflammatory drugs. If the pain is over the inner side of the elbow, gentle stretching exercises of the muscles on the front of the forearm help. Radiohumeral joint injury is another form of pitcher's elbow and gives pain on the outer side but recovery is slow because the joint surfaces themselves are damaged by the forces of the throw.

Little league elbow is the pitcher's elbow of children. The structures on the inner side of the elbow are stressed, but, whereas in adults injuries to the soft tissues occur, in children the soft tissues are stronger than the bone and a piece of bone is pulled off the inner side of the elbow. A child with elbow pain needs to be treated seriously to avoid growth abnormalities. Best treated with RICE. A sling or plaster cast may be needed. If the fragment is large, a reattachment operation may be necessary. Little league elbow takes six weeks to heal, but if an operation is performed it may be many months before the elbow can straighten. Do not push the elbow straight; allow the child to work gradually at his or her own pace. The number of pitches per week needs to be controlled and round-arm throwing (to produce a curved flight of the ball) should be discouraged as it appears to contribute to the injury. Many of these injuries result from poor technique.

Shoulder injuries such as **Shoulder separation, Impingement** (subacromial bursa) are common. The fingers suffer too (**Mallet finger**); fractures of the fingers are common in baseball and softball, as is **Dislocated finger**.

Sliding techniques can be classified into two categories, head-first and feet-first. The younger player or novice should not attempt head-first slides which should be reserved for the more experienced player. A properly executed feet-first slide also requires practice because if the foot gets caught in the playing surface. or the player over-slides the base, injuries can occur.

Basketball/handball/volleyball

Hand injuries occur when catches are mis-timed. They include **Mallet finger, Thumb sprain, Dislocated finger** and fractures of the fingers. A well-timed catch allows you to use the whole of the hand, not just the fingers. The block and grab technique of catching in basketball can prevent many of these injuries. One hand is held up to receive the ball and the other comes around the front to complete the catch. Receiving the ball with both hands puts excessive strain on the back of the thumbs.

Tall players have a high center of gravity, and this makes **Sprained ankle** and **Inner ankle sprain** more common. Some coaches insist on ankle strapping, although others feel this transfers the stress to the knee. **Soccer player's groin** (osteitis pubis symphysis) affects basketball and handball players who tend to back off from the opponent. **Jumper's knee** (patella tendinitis) may occur from jumping for the ball. Catching and throwing the ball above the head can cause shoulder problems such as **Painful arc/rotator cuff rupture** and **Impingement** (subacromial bursa).

Boxing

The majority of injuries in boxing affect the face and head. Head guards are important during training, even if you feel you are superior in skill to your opponent. Mouth guards are mandatory and can be bought ready made, although custom-made guards are much better if you can afford them. In recent years boxing has received bad publicity, and some have tried to ban the sport. Practiced sensibly most severe injuries are avoidable, although minor cuts and bruises are bound to occur. In terms of mortality, the professional boxer is less at risk than a hang-gliding enthusiast or a mountaineer. It is likely, however, that over the next few years rules will be brought in to try to make this a safer sport, such as regular brain scans for professional boxers.

After a knockout, amateur boxers are not allowed to box for a set period of time: first knockout – 28 days; second knockout – 84 days; third knockout – one year. This is to minimize the risk of the condition known as being punch drunk which leads to a gradual deterioration and change in the personality of the boxer caused by damage to the cells of the brain which cannot reform. See also **Concussion/knockout**.

A boxer with **Nearsightedness** is prone to a **Detached retina** because the thin retina is pulled off the back of the eyeball by pressure waves set up when the eye is hit. If you are nearsighted or have a family history of retinal detachment, think twice about taking up boxing and seek the advice of an eye specialist before deciding if it is worth the risk of a reduction of vision or even blindness.

Boxing is the only sport where successfully cutting the opponent's skin can help you win the match. Cuts around the eye may not be severe, but the bleeding can impair vision. Dilute adrenaline solution shuts down the tiny blood vessels in the skin when applied during the fight and this limits bleeding, but pressure and ice are required as soon as possible after the fight. Stitching may be needed to stop bleeding or to prevent a weak scar from developing. Repeated punching may produce boxer's arm, caused by an outgrowth of bone just above the elbow joint where one of the muscles is attached to the bone. The spur can get broken off during a fight causing pain above the elbow. The treatment is rest and the pain usually subsides in four to six weeks after injury.

Canoeing/kayaking

These sports are frequently persued on dangerous reaches of water, so keep within the limits of safety and do not canoe alone. People underestimate the importance of total fitness and good technique. Wear head protection if you are likely to turn over or be in water where there are many boulders such as rapids.

Tenosynovitis of the wrist and **Tennis elbow** are caused by gripping too hard and twisting. Both may respond well to an improved technique. Back pain may develop after prolonged periods of sitting and building up the strength of the abdominal and back muscles may prevent this. The constant kneeling while learning to canoe may cause **Housemaid's knee**, so start sitting as soon as you can manage or use some sort of knee protection. Hypothermia (a dangerous drop in body temperature) can occur in most watersports, particularly in cold weather. Much heat can be lost by water evaporating from your body even if you are not immersed in water, and this is particularly true in windy weather when there may be a high wind chill factor, so dress sensibly in a wet suit, well cut away under the arms with loose sleeves. It is also advisable to wear a life saver.

Cycling

More and more cyclists are now wearing some sort of head protection. Many cyclists have constantly gritty eyes from wind and sun exposure. Although lubricating ointments can give some relief, sunglasses give good protection. The best type are polycarbonate eye protectors. Do not wear sunglasses made of glass.

Prolonged sitting on the saddle can injure the male genitals and occasionally torsion of the testicle (twisting) may occur. It may be possible to untwist the testicle and relieve the pain. However, medical attention should be sought immediately, especially if pain persists, as a delay of even a few hours can lead to permanent sterility. Another embarassing problem is priapism (continual erection of the penis). This may subside once the rider dismounts the cycle, but if the problem persists, medical advice is needed. Priapism is variously thought to be caused by pressure on either the nerves or the blood vessels supplying the penis.

Padding on the handles of the bike may help to prevent **Ulnar neuritis/funny bone** or **Carpal tunnel syndrome** which is caused by constant pressure on the palm of the hands from the handlebars. The structures involved in extending the knee are put under tremendous stress during cycling causing **Quads insertion pull** and **Kneecap pain** (patello-femoral pain syndrome).

Cyclists may get heartburn from leaning forward on the bicycle because exertion raises the pressure within the abdomen and makes the acidic stomach contents reflux up the esophagus causing inflammation. Raising the handlebars may alleviate the problem, or taking an antacid before a race. If symptoms persist, seek medical advice.

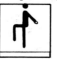

Diving/trampolining

Neck injuries can occur in both these sports if they are not adequately supervised. (See **First Aid: Section Three.**) Such an injury can be devastating causing paraplegia or tetraplegia (paralysis of the limbs), especially when children are taking part unsupervised. A twisting fall onto the trampoline or into the water is dangerous. Good training avoids most of these injuries.

A high velocity dive may cause wrist sprains, thumb sprains and shoulders injuries because of the high impact velocity when the diver hits the water. **Osgood Schlatter's disease** may affect youngsters doing a lot of springboard work.

Trampolining is great fun but potentially dangerous because it is easy to lose control. It has been suggested that it should not be encouraged as a school activity. Two top class adult polevaulters have become paraplegic following injuries during trampolining. The high G-forces may cause momentary loss of consciousness resulting in an awkward fall, so be careful.

Fencing

Faulty equipment can make fencing dangerous. The face mask can become rusty particularly where you are breathing on it, so keep a check.

In hot climates salt and fluid loss may cause weakness and cramp. Salt tablets are not usually necessary as extra salt in the diet is enough. Blisters and skin tears are more common in hot weather. Skin creams help to avoid cracking.

Field Hockey

Like golf, field hockey is played with a bias towards one side and because much of the running is done in an unbalanced position, back injuries and hamstring injuries are relatively common particularly among veteran players who do little in the way of training, so watch out. Warming-up exercises and hamstring stretches are particularly important.

Certain injuries are more common on artificial surfaces, particularly **Soccer player's groin** (osteitis pubis symphysis). High knee hip pain occurs because the player runs in the bent position.

Football

This is a high speed contact sport and injuries are common. It is estimated that some three million people participate annually in the sport, of which 50% will receive some injury during the year. The majority of these will be relatively minor sprains and bruises, however. Due to the nature of the sport, significant injuries to the head, eyes and jaw have been the cause of considerable concern and the basis of legislation for the use of protective face and mouth guards. Unfortunately, although there has been a proven reduction in facial and eye injuries since the introduction of these devices, blocking and tackling techniques have changed and there is a temptation for the player to use his helmeted head as a weapon. This puts the cervical spine at risk. Although these neck injuries are uncommon, their potential severity makes their prevention by strict adherence to the rules extremely important.

Injuries include **Dislocated kneecap** and other knee injuries, **Shoulder separation** (acromio-clavicular dislocation) due to a direct blow, and the less common true **Shoulder dislocation** is also seen. **Dislocated finger** is common.

Low back pain, also common, is caused by

hyperextension of the back. Recurrent episodes of this injury may cause chronic low back pain, and in some cases may permanently injure the bones of the back, causing subsequent instability at the base of the spine (spondylolisthesis).

Golf

If golfers spent a fraction of the time they spent on the 19th green getting fit and staying supple, most golfing injuries would never happen. The typical golfer drives out of town on a Saturday morning after a hard week at the office and goes straight onto the first tee without much of a warm-up. For warm-up exercises see **Section One**, but concentrate on the hip and shoulder swings, particularly in cold weather. Golf is very much a one-sided game which can lead to imbalance in muscle groups. This can be avoided by swinging in the opposite direction at the beginning and end of the game.

Upper back pain and low back pain are both common problems. A smooth, balanced swing and pre-golf exercises can avoid most of these problems, but if back pain persists medical advice is needed. Manipulation or traction can help.

Golfer's/javelin thrower's elbow usually occurs because the player grips the club too hard, or frequently hits the ground. Once the problem arises a period of rest may be all that is required to let it subside. Persistent problems may need ultrasound or cortisone injections.

Tennis elbow arises from a closed right-hand grip without adequate swing, and gripping too tightly or hitting the ground aggravates the condition. Your professional may be able to help you adjust your grip and swing, otherwise treatment is similar to golfer's elbow. Wrist injuries may arise from hitting the ground, but RICE usually settles these within a day or two.

Gymnastics/aerobics

Gymnastics are most successfully practiced by growing girls because they have all the qualities needed for success: short stature, nimbleness, and supple joints and ligaments. However, these very advantages are often a cause of injury.

Sway back elbow is an injury caused by frequent hyperextention (overstraightening) of the elbow. Exercises to strengthen the elbow may give it more stability and prevent pain, but rest may also be required for a period. There is little that the medical profession can offer if this becomes a chronic problem. Repeated injuries interfere with technique and cause the gymnast to use trick movements to get around the problem. These can lead to technical faults which may be dangerous.

Quads mechanism injuries **(Quads insertion pull; Quads muscle pull; Quads injury), Kneecap pain** and **Osgood Schlatter's disease** are common and may be difficult to cure. Early treatment is better than continuing and ending up with a more serious problem. Avoid squatting exercises and work on the bar and beam. Concentrate on arm exercises and suppleness on the floor. Roll out of vaults rather than doing spot landings.

Hyperextension causes back injuries. Posture is not the problem here, but make sure you are warming up adequately. Swimming is a good rehabilitation exercise that does not put a strain on the back.

Stress fractures of the radius (the bone on the outer side of the forearm) affect gymnasts doing the Tsukahara-type jump, twisting on the weight-bearing wrist.

In the past few years, aerobics have become extremely popular as a means of staying fit and toning the body.

Most aerobic injuries occur below the knee and are caused by repeated jumping motions, resulting in **Shin splints**, neuroma (a nerve pain between the toes), **Metatarsalgia** (pain in the ball of the foot), **Stress fracture, sprained ankle** and **Cartilage tears**.

Proper shoes and complete warming up and cooling down exercises are extremely important. It is also advisable to learn not to overdo this form of exercise; use common sense and stop when you are tired or feeling any discomfort.

Handball
See **Basketball/handball/volleyball.**

Horseback riding

Most injuries are caused by falls and the most disasterous are head and neck injuries. The classic type of riding hat is almost useless and much safer, less attractive types are now on the market. (See **Section One: Protective Equipment**.)

The knee is prone to injury from falls resulting in **Lateral ligament strain/rupture**, or fracture of either the lower end of the thigh bone or the upper part of the shin bone. This may be a minor compression (squeezing) of the surface of the joint requiring physical therapy and crutches for six to twelve weeks, or a more severe injury needing surgery with bone grafting and pinning. **Shoulder separation** and **Fractured collarbone** are painful injuries caused by landing on the tip of the shoulder. Refracture can occur with another fall for up to six weeks after the injury, so take care.

Neck injuries need to be handled with great care. If a rider complains of neck pain or tingling, numbness or weakness in any limb, follow the principles laid out in **Section Three: First Aid**.

Bad riding technique results in falls and injuries, so keep your movements smooth. All manner of injuries occur when stepped on or kicked by a horse, some of them severe. Get out of the way if you fall off the horse, and if you cannot, try to curl up in a ball like a hedgehog. Nine times out of ten the horse will manage to avoid you. Remember that horses are dangerous at both ends and uncomfortable in the middle. Don't stand behind a horse, and keep children away unless attended. Horses give nasty bites, particularly on children's faces.

Ice hockey

Most of the injuries in ice hockey are caused by direct impact with the player's stick or puck. Injuries to the face, eyes and teeth are well documented and there are strict rules relating to the use of proper helmets with face guards, which do not allow the penetration of the hockey stick, and the use of these considerably reduces severe facial injuries.

Severe abdominal injuries can be caused by a direct blow from the stick (spearing) which is strictly outlawed. In ice hockey, probably more than any other sport, strict adherence to rules and the use of correct protective clothing makes the avoidance of most injuries possible.

Ice skating

This sport is very dangerous on open water where ice may be thick at the edge, but break under your weight at the center, or where warmer water is flowing into the lake. It is much safer to skate on a rink.

Fractures are more common on ice than ligament injuries. When you fall you tend to slide instead of twist. The most common fractures are a **Fractured radius** and **Fractured scaphoid** of the wrist which come from falling on the outstretched hand. A fall backwards may also cause a head injury (see **Section Three: Treatments**) or **Coccygitis (coccydynia)**. Ill-fitting boots can cause ligament strain or rupture of the ankle, as well as skater's heel where the boot rubs and causes a bursitis (inflammation of the protective fluid-filled sack covering the heelbone). Catch it early and treat with RICE, but more importantly, change your boots. Persistent swelling may need needling to draw off the fluid. Surgery is rarely required.

High knee hip pain is common among speed skaters who tend to bend forwards while they are skating. Figure skaters can suffer from stress fractures because of the jumps, and the tibia (shin bone) is usually the bone to be affected. Try to limit the number of jumps.

Jogging
See **Running/jogging**.

Judo

Remarkably few injuries occur in what to outsiders seems a fairly violent sport, but fractures of the fingers and toes can happen, as can **Cauliflower ear/wrestler's ear**. The mechanism of some injuries is the same as many racquet sports resulting in **Tennis elbow** and **Golfer's/javelin thrower's elbow**. A specilialized splint with a band around the upper part of the forearm may prevent the recurrence of tennis elbow. The forcible straightening of the elbow during an arm-lock can cause more serious injury to the ligaments at the front of the elbow. Nerves and blood vessels may also be damaged if associated with a dislocation at the joint. Seek medical advice or recovery may be prolonged.

Falls need regular practice to avoid **Shoulder separation**. A partial tear of the ligaments of the joint needs sling rest for a few days, but a severe tear may take three weeks before it feels comfortable. Exercises to maintain a good range of movement during rehabilitation are important. **Fractured collarbone** is also caused by a fall on the shoulder and takes three weeks to heal, although a return to the sport is unwise before six weeks. **Shoulder dislocation** may be caused by a fall or a hold and recovery is typically six weeks. Go to the nearest emergency room for urgent treatment if the shoulder does not relocate itself, and do not go straight back to match play. Train on muscle power and make sure you are really fit before attempting too much. **Fractured ribs** do occasionally occur from blows to the chest wall. It is wise to have a physician listen to your chest to ensure that the lung is still inflated, but complications are rare. Strapping is useless. A fractured rib is usually harmless but very painful; coughing and laughing will bring tears to the eyes.

Fluid balance may be a problem particularly in a hot atmosphere when a long match is being played. Take plenty of fluid beforehand – you may need to stock up during the match. It may be worth taking additional salt in the diet in the short term if, for example, you are playing in a hot country.

Kayaking

See **Canoeing/kayaking**.

Motocross/dirt biking

This off-road motorcycling is quickly gaining popularity among youngsters. Although it is potentially dangerous, it is probably a fairly safe way of teaching younger motorcyclists their limitations before they take to the open road. However, children start their scrambling careers younger and younger and the injuries are becoming proportionally more severe. This is partly because the young skeleton is softer than that of an adult, but also because the relative weight and velocity of the motorcycle is higher in the younger age group.

Do not even consider getting on a motorcycle without a helmet – it is madness (see **Section One: Protective Equipment**). Proper protective clothing saves you from most grazes, cuts and bruises. Your jacket may be ruined, but at least you will survive.

The knee is the most common site of injury following collision with other motorcycles or stationery objects. Knee protectors are available and wheel guards prevent the foot from getting caught in the spokes. Back injuries are most common among younger members and are usually caused by a simple fall which overbends the spine. If you suspect a spinal injury, follow the First Aid instructions in **Section Three: Treatments**.

Racquetball

See **Squash/racquetball**.

Rowing

A considerable amount of land training is needed particularly in northern climates where dark winter nights and ice make rowing almost impossible.

Low back pain is common because of the forces taken through the back while in a sitting position. Although rowers have incredibly strong abdominal muscles, the sitting position does not allow these muscles to support the back. (In normal lifting the abdominal muscles and trunk take about one third of the force of the lift.) Many back injuries occur outside the boat during weight training – do more repetitions with lower weights, build up back musclature and work on abdominals with sit-ups.

Upper back pain, often felt as pain in the chest and ribs, is caused by overreaching although sculling on a winding bit of river can cause the problem. Strong back and abdominal muscles prevent this, and manipulation can give dramatically swift relief.

Quads mechanism injuries are common because considerable forces are put through the bent knee. The problem may be traced back to bad training techniques. Rest is often the only answer, then a building up of the muscles with the knee straight. Less compression at front-stops lessens the strain of the structures on the leg. Rowers also suffer from **Tenosynovitis of the wrist** (see **Canoeing/kayaking**) in the hand nearest the oar which is constantly turning. **Blisters** are common at the beginning of the season. Burst them with a sterilized pin rather than letting them rupture while rowing. Seek medical advice if a blister appears to become infected.

Hemorrhoids are a common problem among rowers because of the position adopted. There are various creams on the market which do much to relieve the discomfort of hemorrhoids and a high fibre diet is thought to make hemorrhoids less common. Hemorrhoids are relatively harmless although bleeding may be rather alarming and occasionally quite serious. If hemorrhoids persist, seek medical advice.

Running/jogging

Jogging is a form of running. It has become extremely popular in recent years as an exercise for strengthening the heart, increasing lung capacity, lowering blood pressure, and helping to tone the body by burning calories. Before taking up this form of exercise, however, as in all other sports, it is important to have a complete physical checkup.

The most common problems that may result from running or jogging are **Blisters, Runner's toe, Shin splints, Hamstring sprains,** and **Sprained ankle**.

It is extremely important to have the proper shoes; running shoes that fit well and are specifically designed for running or jogging can prevent many of the injuries mentioned above. (See **Protective Equipment**, page 16.)

It is also advisable to perform warm-up exercises before running or jogging, and to use common sense as to the proper weight of your clothing and your fluid intake, in order to prevent heat exhaustion and dehydration.

Sailing

Sailors should always be prepared for the worst. A beautiful calm water with a fresh wind can quickly turn into a dangerous sea. All boating equipment should be in good condition and ideally everyone in the boat should be able to swim. If not, the life vest he or she wears must give adequate flotation (see **Section One: Protective Equipment**).

Small boat sailing is an energetic sport and does require a degree of fitness. Much of the activity involves isometric muscle exercise (when the muscle is contracting but the limb is static). Isometric exercise may be even more demanding than normal exercise and require a high level of fitness, so training is wise. Work particularly on quads and abdominal muscles.

Hypothermia is the main enemy of the sailor and is responsible for the loss of many lives, so wear sensible clothing. Dehydration can sometimes be a problem, particularly when an excursion is longer than expected; take some drinking water with you. Put on a sunscreen because not only are you subjected to the sun's rays for many hours without shade, but also to rays reflected off the water with an added windburn factor. Pterigium affects sailors. It is a type of fibrous tissue which develops at the inner or outer side of the white of the eye caused by exposure to wind, wind-blown sand, salt spray and sunlight. It is easily avoided by wearing sunglasses, but make sure they are shatterproof.

Shooting

Most injuries are accidental and could be avoided by following the gun code. Always assume a gun is loaded; never point a gun at a person, even in jest; never let a child play with a gun even if you are sure it is not loaded; break the gun before climbing over an obstacle or carrying it in a car; assemble a broken gun by moving stock to barrel so that the barrel is always pointing at the ground.

Housemaid's knee and **Olecranon bursitis** comes from leaning on the elbow and knees, but pads prevent this. Always wear ear muffs to deaden the sound or damage to the tiny bones in the middle ear may lead to premature deafness.

Skiing

One of the most exhilarating sports made safer by improvements in equipment. A few years ago, ankle fractures were common. Ski boots were made longer to compensate, but unfortunately fractures of the tibia (shin bone) became more common. The modern ski boot puts more stress on the knee causing ligament strains or more severe ligament ruptures. They are caused by twisting and bending forces and do not always occur at high speeds. Have your bindings set by the local sports shop where you are skiing because they know about local skiing conditions. If bindings are too tight the ski will not come off when you crash, and you may be injured. If the bindings are too loose the ski will keep coming off when you are turning. However, if in doubt, it is best to play safe and have the binding too loose.

Try to keep your legs together with your weight forward to avoid injury. Quads mechanism injuries can be prevented by avoiding long runs in a crouched position. A torn cartilage may result from a twisting fall. If the skier falls on unyielding snow or ice, injuries such as **Shoulder dislocation, Fractured collarbone** or **Shoulder separation** may occur. Occasionally a skier sustains a head injury (see **Section Three: Treatments**).

Skier's thumb occurs when the thumb is pulled sideways as the skier puts a hand out to save a fall. If this is a simple strain without thumb instability, RICE and strapping is usually adequate treatment. A complete rupture of the ligament usually requires surgery. If you are not sure, seek medical attention as what seems to be a relatively minor injury may cause lasting disability if not treated within a week or so. In 1986 a glove was first introduced which had a web between the thumb and index finger. This type of glove will probably become more widely available.

Fitness is an essential for an enjoyable skiing holiday. Too many people go out untrained and are then surprised when they injure themselves. Fatigue leads to mistakes. Build up the muscles around the knee with regular running. The right equipment is also essential (see **Section One: Protective Equipment**).

Soccer

Adductor muscle strain and **Hamstring sprains** are caused by overstretching sideways or forwards with the leg. Adductor strain is caused by a kick using the inner side of the foot. **Soccer player's groin** (osteitis pubis symphysis) is caused by one-sided kicking or backing off from another player. Quads mechanism injuries are usually caused by bad training practices. **Soccer player's ankle** is due to repeated minor injuries which cause the ankle ligaments to stretch. **Inner ankle sprain, Sprained ankle,** ligament strain and fractures of the fibula are common especially when cleats are used on very hard ground. Knee ligament injuries such as **Lateral ligament strain/rupture, Medial ligament strain/rupture** and **Cartilage ligament injury** occur when the knee of the weight-bearing leg twists. **Fracture of shin bone** (tibia) results from a direct blow on the shin during a front tackle.

Softball

See **Baseball/softball**.

Squash/racquetball

Very popular sports and an excellent way of keeping fit in a short space of time each week. This convenience tends to mean that there are many who play once a week and do no other exercise. Squash and racquetball demand not just stamina, but stretches and turns at speed. It is worth trying to fit in one or two runs per week of perhaps 15 or 20 minutes with some sprints after a warm-up jog. You will avoid injury and probably find the game more enjoyable.

Eye injuries are relatively common because the squash ball fits perfectly into the socket of the eye. An older or more casual player is particularly as risk because of slow reflexes, although with a ball that can travel at up to 100 mph, even those with lightening reflexes can be injured. Protective spectacles are widely available (see **Section One: Protective Equipment**).

Quads mechanism injuries may be a problem on the racquet side of the body. Poorly fitting shoes may result in an **Inner ankle sprain**, a **Sprained ankle, Broken ankle bones** (fracture), **Ligament rupture, Blisters** or **Black nail/runner's toe/turf toe**.

Tennis elbow occurs less frequently than in the tennis player but a faulty technique is often to blame. For example, playing a forehand shot with too closed a grip, or playing a backhand with a dropped racquet head. This can also cause **Pronator teres syndrome**.

Squash player's finger occurs when the player grips the

racquet too hard with the thumb and index finger. Pain is felt at the back of the hand. Adjust your grip so that more of the strain is taken by the other fingers.

Surfing

Surfer's foot is an overgrowth of bone underneath the great toe joint because weight is centered over the instep. Surfer's rub is caused by the rubbing of the wetsuit and can be prevented by applying petroleum jelly or some similar compound to the skin. When the surfer lies on the board, wax may rub off and cause wax rash on the skin. Wearing a T-shirt or wetsuit usually solves this problem and also protects the skin from sunburn. Use a waterproof sunscreen to be on the safe side (See also: **Swimming**).

Swimming

A competent swimmer in safe water is the least likely candidate for a sports injury and swimming is an excellent treatment for many sports injuries. However, chlorine can cause an inflammation of the eye (conjunctivitis). An infection of the stomach (gastroenteritis) can develop if you swallow water contaminated by sewage at the seaside – this is usually attributed to food poisoning.

The only common injury in swimming affects those who swim long distances every week. They get swimmer's shoulder, a combination of **Painful arc/rotator cuff rupture** and **Impingement** (subacromial bursa) from continuous use of the shoulder joint and muscles. Cut down the training distances and work on fitness in the gym with exercises that do not involve a large range of shoulder movement, until the pain subsides.

Breast stroke can strain the ligaments around the knee but a reduction of the width of the leg kick solves this problem. Back strain may develop from butterfly stroke, and a reduction in the training schedule may be necessary.

Tennis

The classic injury is **Tennis elbow** which arises because of technical error in play of the backhand shot. A small racquet head, an overtight grip and half-missed shots aggravate the problem. An open stance for forehand shots puts a tremendous strain on the elbow, as does a heavy or unbalanced racquet, although modern racquets seem much more able to absorb the impact of a fast-moving tennis ball. Remember to keep the racquet head high. Two-handed backhand players rarely get tennis elbow, presumably because there is less strain on the tendons. An injury to the radiohumeral joint (pitcher's elbow) produces the same symptoms as tennis elbow, and the treatment is much the same. **Rigid toe** (hallux rigidus) is aggravated by tennis, and back problems may develop because one side of the body is trained harder than the other.

Trampolining

See **Diving/trampolining**.

Waterskiing

Beginners tend to suffer from low back pain because they lean forward. Regular skiers need to work on back muscles. One very unpleasant injury more likely to occur with beginners who have difficulty standing up, is a high pressure enema when water is forced up the rectum or vagina. It is not only unpleasant, it can also cause severe rupture of the internal organs. Tennis elbow can develop if the tow rope is held horizontally for too long. Bend your elbows and let your biceps do the work.

General safety rules are: never ski in shallow water because in a fall you can collide with the bottom; keep away from swimmers; always have two people in the tow boat, one to drive, the other to watch the skier; never drink and waterski; and wear a life vest even if you are a competent swimmer because you may lose consciousness during a fall.

Weightlifting

A useful way of building muscle strength and power, but bad technique can lead to back injuries. Always keep your back straight. A belt may help by transmitting more of the force through the abdominal wall instead of the back. A hernia (rupture) can occur because of the high pressures that build up within the abdomen during weightlifting. A lump appears in the groin, usually at the same time as a sudden pain in that area. The lump may disappear if you lie down, or get bigger if you cough. This is not a dangerous injury but your doctor may advise you to have an operation to get rid of the lump. If you do have an operation, the surgeon will advise you about getting back to the sport.

Other injuries that can affect weightlifters include **Biceps strain, Shoulder separation** and chest wall pain from injuries of the chest muscles during bench presses. Fainting sometimes occurs because of the high pressure inside the abdomen which prevents blood from returning to the heart and brain. If fainting becomes common, seek medical advice. Do not lift heavy weights when you are pregnant because the hormones of pregnancy slacken the ligaments and injury is more likely.

Windsurfing

Good standards of stamina are required especially in rough weather. Back, thigh and forearm muscles all take a beating, so work on these. Always wear a wetsuit unless you are in tropical waters. Gloves give the hands good protection. You should not take up this sport unless you are a competent swimmer, but even so, always wear a life vest in a bright color.

Bad posture can cause back injuries, and quads mechanism injuries can occur if you are constantly hauling the sail out of the water.

A-Z of Medical Terms

Abscess Infection causing a collection of pus, a boil.

Abdominal Of the abdomen, the area between the base of the rib cage and the pelvis.

A/C joint Stands for acromio-clavicular joint situated at the point of the shoulder at outer end of collarbone.

Adductor muscles Muscles that pull the thigh inward.

Ankle wobble board Balancing board used by physical therapists to improve co-ordination in the legs and to re-educate the muscles after injury, e.g. after ankle sprain.

Anterior Front

Anti-bruise cream Contains an anti-inflammatory to reduce bruising.

Arthritis Damage to shiny surface of joint caused either by disease or injury.

Asthma Wheezing and shortness of breath caused by narrowing of the air passages in the lung. Usually a spontaneous condition in children but may be brought on by exercise or chest infections in some individuals.

Biceps Big muscle at front of upper arm which bends the elbow.

Biceps femoris One of the hamstring muscles on the outer side of the thigh.

Bunion Lump on inner side of the foot at the base of the big toe. Tends to run in families, made worse, but probably not caused by, ill-fitting shoes.

Bursa Normal, fluid-filled sac which lies on top of prominent bones such as at the knee and elbow. It may become inflamed (see BURSITIS).

Bursitis Inflamed bursa, usually caused by overuse giving rise to swelling and pain, as in housemaid's knee and olecranon bursitis of the elbow.

Calcaneum Heel bone.

Capsule Fibrous area around most joints which holds the bones in place to form the joint.

Capsulitis Inflamed capsule.

Cardiovascular system Heart, lungs and blood vessels.

Cartilage 1. Shiny, slippery material that covers the bone ends at a joint allowing the surfaces to glide over each other, known as articular cartilage. This is damaged in arthritis. 2. Half-moon shaped piece of tissue in the knee joint which acts as a shock-absorber between the bones of the thigh and shin. There are two cartilages in each knee. The medical term for this type of cartilage is a meniscus.

Cervical spondylosis Wear and tear arthritis in the small joints in the neck.

Chondromalacia Softening of the shiny cartilage within a joint. Most common in the knees of teenagers.

Clavicle Collarbone.

Compress Bandaging used to hold hot or cold pad firmly against damaged area.

Congenital Inherited.

Contusion Bruise.

Costal Of the ribs.

Crepitus Clicking or grating usually related to joint or tendon.

Cruciate ligaments Pair of crossing ligaments in the knee joint which are important in maintaining joint stability.

Deltoid Muscle at the top of the arm which lifts it at the shoulder.

Dorsiflex Bend upward, as in wrist and ankle.

EMG Electromyography. A test which measures the nerve supply to a muscle.

Epidural Space around the spinal cord and its nerves. The term usually refers to an injection of anesthetic into this space which numbs the nerves in the lower part of the body either for pain relief or for an operation.

Extension Straightening of a joint.

Faradism Application of rapidly alternating electrical current to muscle. Usually used to improve muscle tone and function after injury.

Femur Thigh bone.

Fibula Small bone on outer side of shin bone which forms part of ankle joint.

Flexion Bending of a joint.

Fracture Break in a bone.

Gait Style of walking or running.

Gastrocnemius Big muscle at back of calf.

Hamstrings Big muscles at the back of the thigh which bend knee.

Hematoma Severe bruise with a collection of blood.

Humerus Upper arm bone.

Impingement Abnormal rubbing together of two parts of a joint giving rise to pain, as in a shoulder impingement.

Inflammation Heat, swelling, redness and pain which is the body's reaction to an injury or infection.

Isometric exercise Tightening of a muscle without joint movement.

Laceration Cut.

Lateral Belonging to the outer side.

Ligament Very strong fibrous tissue band which holds bones together at joints.

Lumbago Low back pain.

Manipulation Movement of a joint by physical therapist or doctor to increase the range of movement.

Medial Inner side.

Meniscus See Cartilage.

Metacarpals Bones in the palm of the hand.

Metatarsals Long bones which make up the length of the foot.

Metatarsalgia Metatarsal pain.

Microwave Electrical treatment to heat deep tissues.

Mobilization Movement of joints.

Musculoskeletal Of muscles and bones.

Olecranon Part of the ulna bone of the forearm which forms the tip of the elbow.

Osgood Schlatter's disease Inflammation of the shin bone where the tendon from the kneecap joins it.

Osteochondritis dissicans Fragmentation of a small piece of bone under the shiny cartilage of a joint which may subsequently cause damage to the shiny surface and fall out into the joint as a loose body. Usually occurs in the knee.

Osteoarthritis Wear and tear of a joint.

Orthotics Use of any brace or support in the treatment of musculoskeletal disorders: heel wedge, knee brace, lumbo-sacral corset.

Patella Kneecap.

Pectorals Muscles on front of the chest which bring the arms forward for pushing.

Plantarflex Bend foot downward.

Quadriceps (quads) Large muscles at front of thigh which straighten knee.

Radius One of the two forearm bones lying on the thumbside of the ulna.

Referred pain Trick of the body which can give rise to a sensation of pain in a completely different place from the cause of the pain. Often experienced by children who complain of pain in the knee when the trouble is actually in the hip joint.

Scaphoid Small wrist bone.

Scapula Shoulder blade.

Sciatica Pain felt down the back of the leg into the outer side of the calf and down to the foot, i.e., along the course of the sciatic nerve, and is caused by pressure on the nerve root in the back usually by a slipped disc.

Sesamoid bone Bone lying within a tendon, e.g., kneecap.

Soleus Deep part of calf muscle.

Spondylolisthesis Abnormal shift of one backbone (vertebra) on another due to a failure of the normal bony structure.

Sprain Partial tear of ligaments and capsule of joint.

Sternum Breast bone.

Strain Partial tear of muscle or tendon.

Stress fracture Break in bone which occurs due to overuse as opposed to a single direct injury.

Synovial fluid Oil-like fluid which lubricates joints.

Tendon Fibrous band which attaches muscle to bone.

Tenosynovitis Inflammation of tendon and surrounding sheath.

Tibia Shin bone.

Trauma Injury.

Triceps Muscle at back of upper arm which straightens elbow.

Ulna One of the two forearm bones lying on the little finger side of the radius.

Vertebra Single back bone.

Xiphisternum Lower end of breast bone.

Sports and Women

Specific advantages for women include:
1. Better heat loss during exercise
2. Improved bouyancy in water sports from fat, particularly long-distance swimming
3. Better fat-burning mechanism in endurance sports such as marathon runnning
4. Joint looseness in certain sports such as gymnastics, although this can be a disadvantage in other sports
5. Small stature in some sports such as riding

Specific disadvantages for women include:
1. More fat (25% for women and 15% for men)
2. Wide hips and a lower center of gravity than men
3. Less muscle bulk and strength than men
4. Small stature

The breasts, genitals and womb

Breast pain is more common in sports such as running or jumping where there is repeated movement up and down of the breast. Problems include scratches from bra hooks, allergies to synthetics, and jogger's nipple, caused by the nipple rubbing against the seam of the bra or clothing causing inflammation, infection and pain. Keep any scratches clean to prevent infection setting in, particularly around the nipple. Specifically designed sports bras are now available and features to look for include straps positioned near to the neck so that they do not slip off, a fabric of at least 55% cotton, and a wide band below the breasts or a material which clings to the skin to prevent the bra from riding up.

The female reproductive organs lie deep within the pelvis and injuries involving them are rare. The outer genitals may be damaged by a fall on the balance beam at gymnastics, and although extremely painful at the time and for the next few days, injury is seldom severe. Tears of the vagina can occur from waterskiing without a well-fitting wetsuit.

Pregnancy

Olympic gold medals have been won by pregnant women. During the first three months of pregnancy the womb is protected by the pelvis but after the first three months contact sports should be avoided. Heavy weight training should be avoided during pregnancy and for a few months after birth because hormones loosen the ligaments making injury more likely. There is evidence that women who regularly take part in sport have easier births and fewer Caesareian sections.

Menstrual cycle

This affects different sportswomen in different ways and there is no evidence to suggest that the menstrual cycle has any definite influence on performance. During intense physical training menstruation may become irregular or stop altogether. This is not harmful and once hard training ceases a normal cycle starts again. Absence of periods (amenorrhea) may be an advantage for the sportswoman who suffers from depression, tiredness and irritability just before a period (premenstrual syndrome) or periods pains (dysmenorrhea). Even if the cycle is not disturbed, sport and exercise seems to lessen these problems in most women.

The contraceptive pill

Some sportswomen use the pill to reduce period pains or premenstrual syndrome and because it makes the cycle absolutely predictable. However, the pill increases fluid retention and this may be a disadvantage. If you are going to use the pill, make sure you start it some time before you intend to compete. Many top women athletes use the pill without any problems, but take medical advice before starting.

Anemia

Anemia (too few red blood cells) is common among women because a certain amount of blood is lost every month with menstruation and because women tend to eat food with a lower iron content in an attempt to stay thin. Symptoms of anemia include tiredness, poor performance and breathlessness, often accompanied by heavy periods. It is easily treated with iron supplements so if you think that you are anemic, you should see a doctor for a blood test.

Sex tests

Men are barred from female competition and the organizers of sports carry out a simple sex test either by taking a scraping of cells from the inside of the mouth, or by removing a hair. The chromosomes in the cells are then analyzed. Chromosomes are the chains or proteins which are found in every cell in the body. The X chromosomes look like an X under the microscope, the Y like a Y. Every woman has two X chromosomes, every man has an X and a Y chromosome. At present men do not have to have a sex test.

Index